A SELF HELP BOOK FOR MEN AFTER PRISON

CRAFTED BY SKRIUWER

Copyright © 2024 by Skriuwer.

All rights reserved. No part of this book may be used or reproduced in any form whatsoever without written permission except in the case of brief quotations in critical articles or reviews.

For more information, contact : **kontakt@skriuwer.com** (www.skriuwer.com)

TABLE OF CONTENTS

CHAPTER 1: UNDERSTANDING YOUR STARTING POINT

- Accepting your current reality after release
- Identifying immediate needs: housing, income, emotional well-being
- Recognizing the skills you gained and the power of practical thinking
- Setting boundaries and building a daily check-in routine

CHAPTER 2: FACING REGRET AND MOVING FORWARD

- Defining regret and its impact on self-growth
- Taking responsibility and offering sincere apologies
- Making amends and practicing self-forgiveness
- Turning regret into a motivating force

CHAPTER 3: BUILDING A STRONG SELF-IMAGE

- Understanding self-image and why it matters
- Catching negative self-talk and shifting it to balanced thoughts
- Physical posture, grooming, and daily wins
- Using new habits and skills to boost self-worth

CHAPTER 4: HANDLING ANGER IN HEALTHY WAYS

- Recognizing anger triggers and early signs
- Practical methods: deep breathing, stepping away, or counting
- Replacing harmful reactions with better communication
- Staying calm in tense environments

CHAPTER 5: FINDING A STABLE PLACE TO LIVE

- Types of housing: transitional programs, renting rooms, family options
- Budgeting for rent and deposits
- Handling background checks and building references
- Keeping your home safe and steady for long-term security

CHAPTER 6: CREATING SUPPORT THROUGH FRIENDS AND GROUPS

- Why a support network matters after prison
- Rebuilding old friendships and forming new ones
- Finding role models, mentors, and group support
- Balancing help from family, peers, and professional counselors

CHAPTER 7: GETTING A JOB AND BUILDING WORK SKILLS

- Addressing the record issue in interviews
- Searching for openings and crafting a resume
- Overcoming barriers: limited transport, lack of clothes, negative attitudes
- Retaining a job through punctuality, respect, and adaptability

CHAPTER 8: BUILDING BETTER DAILY ROUTINES

- Why routines matter for structure and stability
- Balancing work, family, and personal needs
- Tools to stay organized: calendars, lists, simple schedules
- Avoiding old habits by filling free time with positive tasks

CHAPTER 9: LOOKING AFTER YOUR PHYSICAL HEALTH

- Simple fitness routines for strength and stress relief
- Eating better on a budget: bulk foods, healthier choices, cooking at home
- Regular checkups, dental and eye care, and dealing with stress
- Staying away from substance use and harmful coping methods

CHAPTER 10: STRENGTHENING RELATIONSHIPS WITH FAMILY AND FRIENDS

- Rebuilding trust through honesty and consistent behavior
- Listening skills and apologies for past wrongs
- Setting boundaries and dealing with conflict
- Finding meaningful ways to reconnect or form new bonds

CHAPTER 11: MANAGING STRESS IN EVERYDAY LIFE

- *Recognizing common stress triggers*
- *Healthy ways to lower stress: breathing, exercise, short breaks*
- *Organizing your day to reduce chaos*
- *Using a balanced mindset to handle life's daily pressures*

CHAPTER 12: DEALING WITH MOMENTS THAT REMIND YOU OF PRISON

- *Understanding triggers and flashbacks*
- *Grounding techniques and relaxation methods*
- *Facing triggers gradually and getting support*
- *Turning negative memories into motivation for staying free*

CHAPTER 13: HANDLING MONEY AND BUILDING A BUDGET

- *Basics of income vs. expenses*
- *Cutting back on costs and avoiding high-risk loans*
- *Paying off fines, setting an emergency fund, and improving credit*
- *Planning for financial security and growth*

CHAPTER 14: SETTING CLEAR GOALS FOR THE FUTURE

- *Why goals matter beyond immediate survival*
- *Breaking big goals into smaller steps*
- *Finding mentors or groups to keep you accountable*
- *Staying flexible and motivated over time*

CHAPTER 15: SPEAKING CLEARLY AND LISTENING WELL

- *Communicating with honesty and respect*
- *Avoiding slang, aggressive tones, and poor listening habits*
- *Handling heated conversations and job interviews*
- *Apologies, setting verbal boundaries, and building confidence*

CHAPTER 16: FINDING PURPOSE IN THE MIDDLE OF CHALLENGES

- Defining personal purpose after prison
- Turning past lessons into a guide for future living
- Balancing personal growth and serving the community
- Staying resilient and hopeful in tough times

CHAPTER 17: IMPROVING YOUR SELF-WORTH

- Understanding the concept of self-worth and why it is often low
- Replacing negative self-talk with balanced thinking
- Identifying strengths and avoiding comparisons
- Building a healthier relationship with yourself

CHAPTER 18: COPING WITH UPS AND DOWNS

- Recognizing life's natural highs and lows
- Marking small victories and managing setbacks
- Staying grounded during successes and handling sudden crises
- Using resilience and safe coping methods for the long term

CHAPTER 19: PLANNING FOR A BETTER FUTURE

- Turning hopes into a structured roadmap
- Setting deadlines, managing resources, and filling skill gaps
- Avoiding old triggers through protective strategies
- Staying motivated by updating plans and adapting to life changes

CHAPTER 20: KEEPING UP YOUR PROGRESS FOR YEARS TO COME

- Seeing personal change as a lifelong process
- Maintaining a routine of self-improvement and good habits
- Protecting mental health, nurturing relationships, and giving back
- Avoiding complacency and planning for major life events in the future

Chapter 1: Understanding Your Starting Point

Coming out of prison can feel confusing. You might have mixed feelings about what happened in your past, and you might not know the best way to go forward. Many people face problems such as finding a place to sleep, dealing with anger, or feeling cut off from others. This first chapter looks at what it means to accept where you are right now. It focuses on why it is important to admit what happened, learn from it, and then decide how to move on.

Admitting the Reality of Your Situation

It is normal to feel lost after release. You might have lost touch with friends and family, or you might feel ashamed. Some men also feel pressure because they want to make up for lost time. The first key step is to be honest about where you stand. This can mean writing down a list of the main challenges you face. For example:

1. **Housing** – Do you have a safe space?
2. **Income** – Do you have a job lined up or a way to earn money?
3. **Emotional Health** – Are there feelings of anger, sadness, or guilt that need to be addressed?
4. **Legal Matters** – Are there any court dates or conditions of release that you must remember?

This list might look daunting, but writing it out can help you see what you are dealing with. Many men try to ignore these problems, hoping they will solve themselves. Unfortunately, ignoring problems can lead to more trouble. Some men might panic and feel the urge to turn back to old ways. It is better to look at the facts calmly.

Taking Stock of Skills

You might think that your prison time set you back in every way, but that is not always true. You may have built skills in prison, such as discipline in routines or learning new trades. Some men learned how to read more, how to follow a schedule better, or how to handle conflict without letting it turn physical. Make a list of the skills you have. Examples could include:

- Ability to follow instructions in a strict environment.
- Willingness to keep going in tough settings.
- Possibly you learned job skills, like carpentry, cooking, or welding.

- You might have gained insight into how anger starts and how to slow it down.

These skills are real. They can help you as you begin your new life. Even if you feel you did not learn much, small things can be turned into strengths. For instance, if you spent time reading law books, you might have learned problem-solving strategies. Or if you spent time in a prison work program, you might have work skills to talk about with potential bosses.

Why Mindset Matters

Many men overlook how powerful their own thoughts can be. If you keep saying, "I will fail again," you might push yourself toward failure without meaning to. If you believe you can make better choices, you can start moving toward those better choices. This is not about being unrealistically positive. Rather, it is about practical thinking. A practical approach might be:

- "I have made mistakes, but I can learn from them."
- "I do not know everything, but I can get help."
- "I may face rejection, but I will keep trying."

These thoughts push you in a productive direction. On the other hand, if you say, "I cannot get a good job with my record," you might give up too soon. Employers value honesty and effort. Some employers even look for people who can bring unique skills and want to turn their lives around. A practical mindset helps you see these chances.

Common Mental Blocks

Right after prison, men may struggle with certain mental blocks:

1. **Feelings of shame** – You might feel unworthy of a better life.
2. **Fear of the unknown** – You might not know what society expects from you now.
3. **Anger** – You might feel bitter about how things happened.
4. **Mistrust** – You might not trust authorities or even old friends.

These blocks can lead to self-sabotage if not handled. The first step in dealing with them is identifying them. Once you know you have shame or anger, you can work on ways to reduce their power. For some, it might help to talk to a counselor or a mentor. For others, it might help to create a personal action plan for day-to-day tasks.

Building a Safety Net for Yourself

It is helpful to set up a personal "safety net." This includes people you can call when you feel stressed or when you feel the urge to do something harmful. It might also include a local community center or a group that helps former inmates. You can also find online communities if that is easier. The point is not to fight every problem alone.

- **Local Support Groups**: Some churches, mosques, or community centers have meetings for men who need advice.
- **Counselors**: If you have access to low-cost or free counselors, they can help you work on anger, guilt, or anxiety.
- **Friends or Family**: Even if your relationships are shaky, look for at least one person who is ready to listen.

A safety net does not make your problems go away, but it can give you breathing room. Instead of throwing yourself into a tough situation alone, you can share your load with people who care. They might not have the perfect answers, but they can keep you from feeling totally alone.

Practical Step: A Personal Check-In Routine

One practical method is to have a daily check-in with yourself. Early in the morning or late at night, ask:

1. **What went right today (or yesterday)?**
2. **What went wrong or felt hard?**
3. **What small step can I do today (or tomorrow) to improve?**

Write these answers in a simple notebook. Doing this every day helps you notice patterns. Maybe you always get upset when you see something that reminds you of prison. Maybe you feel low after talking with certain people. Once you see the pattern, you can think of a plan to handle it. Over time, these notes become a record of your progress.

The Importance of Boundaries

Boundaries help protect your well-being. They can also keep you out of trouble. For instance, if you know certain neighborhoods lead you back to old bad habits, stay away. If certain friends always want you to do illegal things, limit your contact with them. If certain topics make you lose your temper, practice stepping away from those discussions.

These boundaries are for you. They are a kind of rulebook that helps you stay clear of traps. You do not have to explain them to everyone. If someone pushes you to do something you do not want, firmly say no. If that person does not respect you, consider whether that person belongs in your life right now.

Analyzing Long-Term Effects

Many people come out of prison with a sense of having lost valuable time. They also wonder how their record will affect them in the long run. These are serious concerns. Yet it is helpful to remember that you can still shape your future. You might need to check in with parole officers, follow certain rules, or do regular tests. These can be frustrating, but try to see them as steps that keep you on the right track.

If you face rejection when applying for jobs or housing, remember that each "no" is not a final verdict on your life. There are men who received many "no" answers but kept looking until they found someone willing to give them a chance. You only need one "yes" to start moving forward.

Why Change Can Be Hard

Changing your life after prison is not just about new habits. It is also about dealing with old mental habits. You might have old thoughts telling you to do things the same way you did before. Or you might have impulses that made sense inside prison but cause trouble outside. For example, in prison you might have needed to be very cautious around others to stay safe. Outside, being too guarded can make it hard to form trusting friendships.

Recognizing that prison life is different from life outside is vital. Be patient with yourself. You are in new territory now. Learn the "unwritten rules" of life outside, such as being on time for job interviews, speaking politely to store clerks, and making an effort to manage your frustrations without shouting or threatening.

Self-Education and Ongoing Learning

You might think you are done with learning, but that is never the case. Continual learning can improve your life in big ways. If you do not have a high school diploma, look into a GED program or adult education classes. If you do not have work skills, search for vocational training programs. If you have internet access, there are many free websites that teach basic computer skills, writing, math, and more.

Many men who come out of prison find that learning a trade or skill opens up doors that were closed before. Even learning how to write a better resume or how to speak in a professional way during interviews can help you land a job you did not think was possible.

Avoiding Self-Sabotage

Self-sabotage happens when you destroy your progress without realizing it. It might look like missing important meetings or snapping at people who try to help. Sometimes it is caused by the belief that you are not worth a better life. If you catch yourself doing something that blocks your own success, pause and figure out why. Are you scared of success because you have never experienced it? Are you trying to punish yourself for past mistakes?

This reflection might be hard, but it is one of the most useful things you can do. Once you understand why you sabotage yourself, you can prepare solutions. For instance, if you skip job interviews because you feel unqualified, remind yourself that you have skills. Practice your interview answers with a friend. This small preparation can lower your fears and keep you from missing the interview.

Defining Your Own Values

Everyone has personal values that guide them. After prison, some men rediscover or redefine what they care about most. Your values might be honesty, hard work, fairness, loyalty to family, or serving your community. When you define these values and keep them in mind, they guide your choices. If your top value is honesty, you will be less likely to lie on an application. If your top value is fairness, you will treat people in ways that match that sense of fairness.

These values can also help you pick friends who respect the same things. This reduces the chance of returning to the bad influences that contributed to your time in prison.

Conclusion of Chapter 1

Understanding where you stand right after prison is the first major step. Be clear about the challenges and also about the strengths you have. Build a personal safety net so you do not face everything alone. Keep track of your progress with a daily check-in. Learn to set boundaries. Recognize your self-sabotaging habits and address them. Know your personal values so you can base your life on what truly matters to you.

Life after prison can be tough, but it is not impossible to overcome obstacles. This first chapter sets the stage for the rest of the book, showing you that there is a structured way to approach each aspect of rebuilding your life. By admitting where you are and preparing step by step, you give yourself a real shot at something better.

Chapter 2: Facing Regret and Moving Forward

Regret is a normal feeling for men who have been to prison. You might regret the crime, the harm done to others, or the impact on your family. You might regret losing years of your life. These feelings can be strong, and if they are not handled well, they can hold you back. This chapter focuses on how to handle regret in a practical way, so it does not block your growth.

Understanding the Nature of Regret

Regret can sometimes cause a person to:

- **Feel hopeless**: "I ruined my life forever."
- **Overthink past mistakes**: "I should have done this differently, but now it is too late."
- **Feel angry at themselves**: "I hate what I did. I cannot forgive myself."

While it is good to admit wrongdoing or failure, getting stuck in regret does not help you or anyone else. It is like staring at a closed door for hours instead of looking for a new door that might be open. A part of regret can be useful because it reminds us not to repeat our mistakes. The trick is to balance that reminder with action toward better living.

Methods to Address Regret

1. **Take Responsibility in Words**
   You might start by clearly stating what you regret. Write it down or say it out loud in a private space. For instance, "I regret hurting that person," or "I regret letting my family down." By putting your regret into clear words, you face it head-on. This stops you from trying to push it away or pretend it never happened.
2. **Apology (If Possible)**
   Sometimes, you might be able to apologize to the people you hurt. This depends on the situation. If it is safe and allowed, you might write a letter or speak to them. The main point of the apology should be honesty. Do not make excuses. Even if they choose not to forgive you, you have taken a step to own your actions.
3. **Find Ways to Make Amends**
   In some cases, you cannot directly fix the harm done. But you can do positive things in your life or community as a sign that you want to change. This could be volunteering, helping your family members with

tasks, or guiding younger people so they do not make the same mistakes. Making amends is about showing, not just telling, that you regret your past.
4. **Self-Forgiveness**
This is often the hardest part. You might feel that you do not deserve forgiveness. Or you might fear that if you forgive yourself, you will forget your wrongdoing. Self-forgiveness is not about forgetting. It is about accepting that you are more than your bad choice. You are a person who can learn. You can continue to carry a sense of responsibility without letting it crush you.

Long-Term Effects of Regret

If regret remains unprocessed, it can turn into bitterness or deep shame. Bitterness may lead you to blame others for your problems. Shame may lead you to hide from people who care about you. Both bitterness and shame can push you back into dangerous patterns, such as substance use or aggression. In the long term, regret needs to be turned into something more productive. Think about how you can learn from your past mistake every day without letting it destroy your sense of self.

The Role of Outside Help

Dealing with regret can be stressful. Sometimes, professional counseling or a trusted mentor can be a big help. You might wonder how a counselor can help if you cannot change the past. Their role is to guide you through the process of sorting out your feelings and building healthier coping strategies. They can give you tools to handle the guilt that creeps in during quiet moments. Sometimes, just talking to a non-judgmental listener can relieve the weight on your shoulders.

Building New Habits to Replace Old Ones

If your regret is connected to a cycle of bad habits—like substance use, theft, or aggression—then building new habits is key. For example, if your old pattern was to get angry and lash out at people, you can replace that with a new habit of taking a few deep breaths and leaving the room to cool down. If your old habit was to hang out with people who led you into crime, you can limit contact with them and seek out more positive people or activities.

Habit change is not always easy. It takes discipline and patience. But each new habit you build helps to reduce the chance of slipping back into the actions you regret. Over time, you might notice that you do not even want those old patterns.

Learning from Mistakes

It sounds simple, but learning from your mistakes is often overlooked. Some people keep feeling guilty but never figure out how to avoid repeating the same error. Take time to reflect on why you made that choice in the first place. Were you in need of money? Were you addicted to substances? Did you have a hot temper? Once you understand the root cause, work on fixing it. This is what true learning from mistakes looks like.

Practical Exercise: Regret Examination

1. **Write down the event or behavior you regret the most.**
2. **Identify who was hurt by it.** Could be yourself, family, friends, or strangers.
3. **Note how it changed your life** – Lost trust, wasted years, legal problems, etc.
4. **Think about what you could have done differently.** This is not to torture yourself, but to learn.
5. **Write down one step** you can take now that would have made sense back then. For instance, if you fell into crime because you felt alone, your step now could be to find a supportive friend or group.

By doing this exercise, you move from just feeling regret to taking an educational look at it. You gain clarity on how to handle similar situations in the present or future.

Handling Self-Criticism

People who feel regret often speak harshly to themselves. They use words like "fool," "loser," or worse. This kind of self-talk does not improve anything. Instead, it feeds a cycle of low self-esteem. Low self-esteem can lead to more mistakes. Try replacing those put-downs with statements that still own the mistake but do not destroy your self-worth. For example:

- **Harsh**: "I am the worst person. I do not deserve another chance."
- **Better**: "I made a harmful choice. I can make better choices now."

This shift in language might feel odd at first, but it matters. You are not lying to yourself; you are recognizing the past mistake and also giving yourself room to move forward.

Interacting with Those You Harmed

Not everyone will welcome you back. Some of the people you harmed might still be angry or scared. Do not force forgiveness or closeness. If they are open to speaking with you, keep your words honest and direct. Let them see through your actions that you are working to live in a better way. If they want no contact, respect that boundary. With time, some of them might change their minds, but you should not push.

When Family Members Are Hurt

Family members can carry deep wounds. They might feel shame that their son, husband, or father ended up in prison. They might have struggled financially or emotionally in your absence. If you want to earn back their trust, you need to show consistent respect and support. For instance, if you promise to help around the house or look for a job, follow through. Words matter, but actions speak louder.

Using Regret as Motivation

Regret can be turned into a type of motivation. For example, if you regret dropping out of school, use that feeling to push yourself to continue your education. If you regret hurting someone, use that as drive to treat people with kindness now. Each time you feel a pang of regret, remind yourself that you are not letting that regret go to waste. You are turning it into a positive push.

It can also be a wake-up call. If you find yourself on the brink of a poor decision, you might remember how regret felt. That memory can help you stop yourself.

The Ripple Effect of Your Actions

Your change in behavior can have a ripple effect on others. Maybe a younger brother who looked up to you sees you working to change and decides to straighten out his own life. Or maybe a friend who was also involved in crime notices your progress and asks you for advice. You cannot erase your past, but you can become a source of constructive influence now. This does not happen overnight, but even small steps can show others that change is possible.

Handling Big Regrets That Cannot Be Fixed

Sometimes, the harm caused is permanent. This might be the hardest situation to handle because you cannot undo the damage. In these cases, the best approach is to fully accept what happened and channel that pain into living in a way that honors the person you harmed or the life you damaged. That might include donating your time to a cause they cared about, or guiding other at-risk individuals away from the same choice you made.

There is no easy fix for large regrets. But by living better each day, you create a small positive mark in the world that offsets a bit of the harm done.

Staying Away from Quick Escapes

When regret hurts, some men look for ways to numb it—through drinking, drug use, or other risky behavior. These quick escapes only push the problem away for a short time. Then the regret and guilt come back stronger. If you notice yourself seeking escape, pause. Acknowledge the pain and consider a healthier coping method. This might be talking to a friend, going for a walk, doing some exercise, or writing down your thoughts. Over time, these healthier methods become your go-to options instead of destructive escapes.

Regret and Hope

It might sound odd to talk about regret and hope together, but they can exist side by side. You can hold regret for your past actions and still have hope for a better future. Hope does not erase guilt or sorrow. It simply points you to the possibility of a brighter tomorrow. Having hope does not mean you pretend the past never happened. It means you refuse to let the past define everything about you.

Conclusion of Chapter 2

Facing regret is important because it can weigh you down if left unchecked. Accepting what you have done, apologizing where you can, and taking steps to make up for it can help you move forward in a better way. Self-forgiveness does not mean you ignore your guilt. It means you stop letting it destroy your ability to change.

Through a combination of honesty, self-reflection, and positive action, you can transform regret into something that pushes you to live better. The chapters to come will cover other aspects of rebuilding life after prison, including anger management, finding a place to live, and building healthy support systems. But keep in mind, dealing with regret is one of the key foundations. Without this step, it is easy to fall back into old patterns.

You have the power to shape a future that is not defined only by your mistakes. Yes, the past is part of your story, but it does not have to be the end of it. By facing regret honestly and turning it into motivation, you free yourself to use your time and energy on building a more stable and productive life.

Chapter 3: Building a Strong Self-Image

Many men who leave prison have a hard time seeing themselves in a good light. They may feel shame about their past or doubt that they can do well in the future. This chapter looks at how to build a solid self-image when life has not always been kind. A strong self-image does not mean being arrogant. It means having a balanced view of who you are—knowing both your good sides and your weak spots, yet still believing you have worth and the ability to move forward.

What Is Self-Image?

Self-image is the idea you have of yourself in your mind. It is like an internal picture you carry all day long. This picture may include how you look, what skills you have, and how much you feel you matter. A self-image can be positive, negative, or somewhere in between:

- **Positive self-image**: "I am capable of learning, and I can do useful things."
- **Negative self-image**: "I am useless and will never achieve anything."

A healthy self-image is not about ignoring past mistakes. Instead, it is about seeing that you have value as a person right now, while staying aware of the areas where you need to grow.

Why a Strong Self-Image Matters After Prison

People who come out of prison often carry the weight of labels. Some may call you an "ex-offender" or other hurtful terms. After hearing such words for a while, you might start believing them. This can lead to hopelessness, which in turn can lead you back into bad choices.

When you work on a healthier self-image, you give yourself a firm base to stand on. Even if others doubt you, your inner sense of worth can keep you going. This does not mean you hide your record. It means you balance it by knowing you can also do good things if you set your mind to it.

Spotting Negative Self-Talk

We all have an internal voice that comments on everything we do. This voice can either lift us up or tear us down. Negative self-talk includes statements like:

- "I am a failure."
- "No one wants me around."
- "I will never be as good as others."

These thoughts might come and go quickly, so you might not even notice them. But they shape how you see yourself. The first step is to identify these thoughts. Pay attention when they pop up. Write them down if possible. Look for patterns. Maybe you feel worthless when you meet someone who has a stable life. Maybe you feel stupid when you cannot do something right away.

Once you spot the negative talk, replace it with balanced thoughts:

- "I made a mistake, but I can learn from it."
- "I might not have all the skills yet, but I can improve over time."
- "I have faced bigger challenges before, and I made it through."

You are not lying to yourself. You are choosing to see the situation in a way that allows you to grow instead of sinking deeper.

The Power of Physical Posture

A simple but often overlooked tip: how you hold your body can affect how you think about yourself. If you slump your shoulders and stare at the ground, you may feel weaker or less sure of yourself. If you stand straight, keep your head up, and look people in the eye, you might notice a bit more steadiness.

Try a small experiment. Stand or sit up straight for a minute or two, breathe evenly, and keep your head level. Notice how this feels in your body. Some men find it helps them speak more clearly and feel more at ease in stressful moments. This tip can be used anywhere—job interviews, family gatherings, or even regular errands.

Dress and Grooming Tips

Clothes do not make the man, but they can affect how you see yourself. After prison, you might not have much money. Still, you can keep your clothes clean and neat. Small steps, like washing your shirt, making sure your jeans are not ripped, and cleaning your shoes, can change how you feel about yourself. Good grooming habits—such as regular showers, trimmed nails, and a basic haircut—show that you respect yourself. You do not need expensive brands or fancy styles. Being clean and tidy is enough to give you a boost of self-confidence.

If you have an important appointment, such as a job interview, see if any local groups or community centers offer help with clothing. Some places donate suits or nice work outfits to men trying to rebuild their lives. Even if you cannot find this kind of help, do the best you can with what you have. Feeling clean and put together can help you hold your head up when you walk into new settings.

Setting Achievable Targets

Another way to build a stronger self-image is by setting small targets and meeting them. These can be daily tasks like:

- Getting up at a set time every morning.
- Cleaning a certain part of your home or living space.
- Spending 15 minutes reading a helpful book or article.
- Practicing a skill for 10 minutes.

Each time you complete a small goal, you get a feeling of success. Over weeks or months, these tiny successes add up. You start seeing yourself as someone who can finish tasks instead of someone who fails. Begin with small steps because they are easier to manage. When you get used to meeting small goals, you can stretch yourself a bit further.

Finding Role Models

A role model is someone you look up to. This does not mean they have to be famous or rich. It could be a neighbor who avoided crime despite living in a tough neighborhood. It could be an older man at a community center who is kind to everyone. A role model shows you that better behavior is possible.

Be careful not to worship someone blindly. Everyone has flaws. Still, you can learn from the good habits they show—things like consistent work, clear communication, or staying calm under pressure. You might even ask them for tips. Some people are happy to share advice, while others lead by example. Either way, having a living example of improvement can help you believe in your own potential.

Handling Criticism from Others

After prison, you may face criticism. Potential employers might be wary of your record. Friends or relatives could doubt your ability to stay on track. Random folks may treat you differently if they learn about your past. This type of judgment can harm your self-image if you let it sink too deep.

Try to separate helpful feedback from hurtful words. If someone says, "You will never amount to anything," that is not helpful. But if a person says, "You need to manage your temper better," that could be valuable advice. Figure out how to tell the difference between shaming language and guidance that can help you grow. Use the helpful tips to improve yourself and let the hateful words go.

Building a Record of Wins

Keep track of your "wins," even if they seem small. You could do this in a notebook or a file on your phone. Wins might be:

- Waking up on time five days in a row.
- Sticking to your budget for the week.
- Learning a new recipe and making it well.
- Staying calm when someone tried to make you angry.

Listing these wins weekly or monthly reminds you that you are getting better, step by step. Men who struggle with self-image often forget their victories. By writing them down, you build a list of clear evidence that you are indeed moving forward.

Correcting Mistakes Without Tearing Yourself Down

You will slip up. Everyone does. The key is how you handle those moments. A man with a shaky self-image might say, "I messed up again, so I must be worthless." A person building a healthier self-image might say, "I messed up, but let me figure out why so I do not do it again."

Try using a simple three-question method after you make a mistake:

1. **What did I do wrong?**
2. **Why did I do it?** (For example, "I was tired," or "I acted out of habit," or "I got angry too fast.")
3. **What can I do differently next time?**

Then forgive yourself and move on. This does not mean you ignore the error. You accept it, learn from it, and keep going.

Building Skills to Lift Your Self-Image

Skills are powerful. They let you see that you can do something useful. Examples include learning a trade such as carpentry or plumbing, picking up computer basics, or improving your reading and writing. Each new skill you gain boosts your confidence.

- **Pick a skill that interests you**: If you enjoy hands-on tasks, look into mechanical or construction areas. If you like talking, you could try public speaking or sales.
- **Find resources**: Community centers, libraries, and online sites often offer free lessons or guides.
- **Track your progress**: Note improvements over time. Even small steps matter.

As you gain skills, you stop seeing yourself only as "the guy with a record." You start seeing yourself as someone with talents.

Staying Around Positive Influences

The people and places around you can shape how you feel about yourself. If you are surrounded by individuals who promote crime or negativity, you may find it harder to believe in your positive aims. If you are often in places that remind you of old habits, you might slip back into them.

Look for people and settings that support your new goals. That could be a local group that focuses on honest living, a sports league that brings people together, or a faith-based gathering if that suits you. You do not have to agree with everyone there, but being in a place where people are trying to improve themselves can have a big effect on you.

The Link Between Self-Image and Physical Health

Your body and mind are connected. Poor sleep, bad eating habits, and no exercise can bring your mood down. Taking care of your health can boost how you see yourself. You do not have to become a fitness expert. Simple changes can help:

- **Aim for 7–8 hours of sleep** if possible.
- **Eat better**: Even on a tight budget, try including fruits, vegetables, and protein in your meals.
- **Move around**: Take walks, do a few push-ups, or stretch at home.

A healthier body often leads to a clearer mind. Feeling more in control of your physical well-being can help your sense of worth.

Taking Ownership of Your Story

Your past is part of who you are, but you decide how the next chapter looks. People might want to define you by your worst moment. You do not have to go along with that. You can accept what happened and still choose to shape your future.

Practice telling your story in a direct, truthful way. For example, if someone asks, "Why were you in prison?" you could say, "I made poor choices that broke the law, but I have been working on turning that around, and I am making progress."

This kind of statement shows you are not hiding, and it also shows you have an eye on the future.

Helping Others to See Your Own Value

Sometimes, the best way to see your worth is to help someone else. Maybe you show a younger person how to handle conflict without using fists. Or you volunteer at a local food bank. You might even help a neighbor with home repairs. When you make a positive difference in someone's day, you are reminded of your ability to do good.

This does not mean overextending yourself. You do not have to save everyone. Even small acts of kindness can change how you feel about yourself. Over time, you will see that you have something valuable to offer the world.

Dealing with Setbacks in Self-Image

No matter how hard you work, there will be days when you feel your self-image slip. Maybe you get a job rejection, or someone from your past says something hurtful. You might think, "All my efforts were pointless." That is when you need to use your tools:

1. **Look at your list of wins.**
2. **Check your self-talk.** Are you slipping back into "I am worthless" talk?
3. **Reach out to your support network.** A phone call or conversation with someone who respects you can help.

A setback is not the end. It is just a moment. The more you practice bouncing back, the more stable your self-image becomes.

Avoid Comparing Yourself to Others

Comparing yourself to people who seem to have it all together is a quick route to feeling bad. Remember that everyone has a different life story. Some have had more support than you did. Some might have faced other challenges you do not see. Focus on comparing yourself to your own past self. Are you doing better than last month or last year? That is progress worth celebrating.

By keeping your eyes on your personal path, you avoid the trap of envy or hopelessness. Your gains may be small, but they are real.

Using Available Resources

These days, there are many free or low-cost resources to help you build a better sense of self. Local community centers might offer workshops on resume writing, anger control, or job skills. Libraries often have free internet access where you can watch helpful videos or do online courses. A simple search can reveal websites with step-by-step guides on everything from budgeting to speaking better in public.

The important idea is to keep learning. You are not stuck in the same self-image forever. Each new piece of knowledge or skill can change how you view yourself.

Staying True to Honest Behavior

A strong self-image is easier to keep if you know you are living with honesty. If you slip into shady dealings or old habits, your sense of guilt might grow, hurting your self-image. Doing what is right, even when no one is looking, builds a sense of personal integrity. It does not mean you are perfect. It means you are trying to live straight. Over time, honest living gives you peace of mind. Peace of mind strengthens how you see yourself.

Practical Steps to Start Building Self-Image

1. **Notebook of Strengths**: Write down three things you did well each day. They can be small, like cooking a decent meal or washing all your clothes.
2. **Daily Target**: Pick a small goal each morning that you know you can complete by night.
3. **Skill Practice**: Spend 15 minutes a day reading or practicing something that improves you.

4. **Mind Your Body**: Drink water, eat nutritious food, and move your body with simple exercises.
5. **Watch Your Words**: If you catch yourself saying, "I can't," swap it with "I will try."

Do these for a week and see how your view of yourself begins to shift.

Conclusion of Chapter 3

Building a strong self-image after prison is a major step in rebuilding your life. It involves noticing negative thoughts, developing positive habits, seeking good influences, and being kind to yourself when you slip. You do not have to pretend your past never happened. Instead, you learn to see yourself as someone who can grow and contribute.

A stable self-image makes it easier to handle struggles, whether they are about finding work, dealing with old friends, or facing new challenges. Other people might still judge you, but if you have a firm belief in your own worth, you will not be swayed by every negative comment. Over time, each new skill learned, each small target met, and each honest action taken will remind you that you are more than your past.

Chapter 4: Handling Anger in Healthy Ways

Anger is a common emotion. Everyone feels it at some point. For men leaving prison, anger can be a serious hurdle. It may come from feeling misunderstood, facing unfairness, or living under stress. In prison, some men had to stay on guard or adopt a tough shell just to survive. That habit can follow them outside, making them quick to lash out or get into fights.

This chapter focuses on practical ways to handle anger without hurting yourself or others. It will not tell you never to feel anger. Instead, it will show you that anger can be handled in a better way, so it does not push you back into bad decisions.

Understanding the Roots of Anger

Anger often has deeper causes. It might come from:

1. **Fear**: Feeling like you could be attacked or disrespected.
2. **Shame**: Being reminded of mistakes or feeling looked down upon.
3. **Frustration**: Wanting something but not being able to get it.
4. **Feeling Powerless**: Believing that life is unfair and you cannot change it.

These roots can mix together. You might feel angry at someone's words, but the real cause might be fear of being judged. Or you might feel rage when you see others succeed because deep down, you feel you are behind in life. Once you identify the root, you can better address the real issue.

Why Anger Control Is Important After Prison

When you have a criminal record, people may already be watching you more closely. If you show anger in unhealthy ways—yelling, threatening, or using force—you risk scaring away potential employers, landlords, or supporters. You could also end up violating the conditions of your release. That might send you back to prison.

Handling anger in healthy ways shows the world that you are serious about change. It also makes your daily life smoother. You avoid fights, keep stress lower, and reduce the odds of making choices you will regret.

Recognizing Anger Triggers

A "trigger" is a person, place, situation, or memory that sparks a strong emotion. Identifying your triggers helps you prepare. Some common triggers might be:

- Being in a crowded space where you feel cramped, similar to prison conditions.
- Arguing about money.
- Feeling that someone is not respecting your personal space.
- A certain tone of voice that reminds you of authority figures who treated you badly.

Triggers differ from person to person. You might try writing them down. Once you see the list, you can plan ways to respond before you lose control. For instance, if you know big crowds make you nervous, you can pick times to shop when stores are less busy. Or you can practice a calming trick before entering a packed bus or waiting room.

The Warning Signs of Anger

Anger often grows step by step. You might notice some signs before you hit full rage:

- Increased heart rate or feeling hot.
- Clenched jaw or fists.
- Shallow or faster breathing.
- A desire to yell or lash out.

Recognizing these signs early is crucial. If you can catch anger at the lower levels, you can calm yourself before it explodes. For example, if your heart is pounding and your teeth are clenched, that is a sign you need to step away or use a calming method.

Simple Calming Methods

1. **Deep Breathing**: Take a slow breath in for a count of four, hold for a second, and breathe out for a count of four. Repeat this a few times. This sends a signal to your brain that you are trying to settle down.
2. **Count Backwards**: Count backward from 10 or even 20. Focus on the numbers rather than the trigger. This brief pause can help you move from instinct to thought.
3. **Leave the Room**: If possible, remove yourself from the situation. Go for a short walk. This is not running away—it is creating space to calm down.
4. **Splash Water on Your Face**: The sudden change in temperature can shift your focus.
5. **Hold Something Cold**: Holding a cold can of soda or pressing an ice cube on your wrist can also help you shift out of the boiling anger feeling.

These methods might sound too simple, but they can be powerful in the heat of the moment. The key is to do them early, before the anger escalates.

Replacing Harmful Reactions with Better Ones

If your old reaction to anger was yelling, making threats, or using force, you need to replace that with a different response. Some ideas include:

- **Verbalizing Calmly**: Say, "I am feeling angry right now. I need a moment." It might feel strange at first, but it gives people around you a warning that you are close to your limit.
- **Writing it Down**: If you cannot speak calmly, step away and write what you are feeling. Sometimes putting words on paper helps cool your thoughts.
- **Seeking a Trusted Friend**: If you have someone in your support circle, call or message them and say, "I am angry about something. Can I talk about it?"

These new reactions take practice. You will not master them in a day. But every time you choose not to react in the old harmful way, you are retraining your mind.

The Role of Exercise

Physical activity is one of the best outlets for anger. Running, boxing, or even brisk walking can release tension. When you exercise, your body burns off some of the stress chemicals that build up when you are mad. This does not fix the cause of the anger, but it helps your body calm down so you can think more clearly.

If you enjoy strength training, you can do push-ups or lift weights. If you prefer something more relaxed, you can do stretching or slow breathing exercises. The goal is not to become a champion athlete; it is to find a physical way to let out the pressure that anger creates inside you.

Talking to a Counselor or Group

Many men avoid counseling because they think it is only for people who are "weak" or "crazy." That is a misunderstanding. Counseling can be very helpful, especially if you have a short fuse. A counselor can teach you methods for handling anger and help you see patterns that set you off.

Group sessions are another option. Sometimes, hearing others talk about their anger struggles can make you feel less alone. You might pick up new tricks or share your own. Some community centers and organizations have free or low-cost anger management groups. If you have a probation officer or social worker, you can ask them for referrals.

Anger and Substance Use

Substances like alcohol or drugs can make anger worse. Some men use substances to escape stress, but these substances lower self-control. That can lead to explosive outbursts. If you already have an issue with anger, adding substances to the mix can cause major problems.

Try to be honest with yourself. If you notice that you often get into fights or arguments while under the influence, it might be time to cut back or stop using those substances. You can look for support groups that deal with both substance issues and anger. Combining help for both can lead to better results than trying to fix them one at a time.

Apologizing When Needed

Everyone makes mistakes, and everyone says or does things in anger they later regret. Learning to say "I'm sorry" shows growth. The apology should be clear and sincere. For example, "I apologize for shouting at you. It was wrong, and I will try to handle my anger better next time."

Apologizing does not make you weak. It shows self-awareness and respect for the other person. This can help repair relationships or at least show people you are serious about changing your ways.

Long-Term Effects of Poor Anger Control

If you do not address your anger problems, you may face serious consequences:

- Loss of relationships: Friends and family might drift away.
- Trouble with the law: Angry outbursts can lead to new charges or parole violations.
- Worsening health: Chronic anger can lead to high blood pressure, headaches, or other stress-related illnesses.
- Missed opportunities: Employers might not want to hire someone with a reputation for being "hot-headed."

On the flip side, controlling your anger can open doors. People see you as reliable and calm under pressure. Your loved ones feel safer around you. You can tackle challenges with a clearer mind.

Anger vs. Assertiveness

There is a big difference between anger and assertiveness. Anger is often emotional and can be aggressive. Assertiveness, on the other hand, is standing up for yourself in a calm, direct way. It means respecting your own needs without trampling on others.

For example, if someone is speaking to you rudely, an angry response would be to yell or threaten them. An assertive response would be to look them in the eye and say, "I do not appreciate being spoken to in that tone. Let's keep this conversation respectful." This sets a boundary without blowing up. Assertiveness helps you keep your dignity while handling conflict in a healthier manner.

Anger and Communication Skills

A lot of anger problems come from poor communication. You might feel like people do not understand you, or you might feel you cannot express your thoughts well. Learning basic communication skills can reduce anger:

1. **Active Listening**: Listen carefully when someone else talks. Do not just wait for your turn to speak. Show you hear them by repeating key points.
2. **Using "I" Statements**: Say, "I feel upset when this happens," instead of, "You make me mad all the time!" This focuses on your feelings rather than blaming the other person.
3. **Avoiding Accusations**: Starting sentences with "You always…" or "You never…" puts people on the defensive. Instead, stick to the specific behavior that bothered you.

These small changes can calm a tense situation because you are not pouring gas on the fire.

Anger and Past Trauma

Sometimes, anger is linked to deep hurt from childhood or past events. Men who were abused or neglected might develop angry reactions as a shield. If you suspect your anger has roots in something that happened long ago, consider speaking to a counselor who specializes in trauma. It can be tough to revisit painful memories, but understanding them can free you from carrying that pain into every argument or misunderstanding.

Practical Exercise: Anger Journal

One helpful tool is keeping an "Anger Journal" for a couple of weeks:

1. **Situation**: Write down what sparked your anger.
2. **Feelings**: Note the emotions you felt—fear, shame, frustration, etc.

3. **Reaction**: Describe what you did—yelled, slammed a door, or walked away.
4. **Outcome**: Note the result. Did it help or hurt the situation?
5. **Alternate Response**: Think of a calmer way you could have handled it.

Review your notes every few days. Look for patterns. You might find the same triggers come up again and again. This insight helps you plan better responses in the future.

Knowing When to Walk Away

There are times when the best move is to remove yourself from the situation entirely. If you are dealing with someone who is trying to provoke you, it is smart to leave. You do not have to stay in a heated argument just because the other person is pushing your buttons. Walking away is not losing. It is choosing to keep yourself out of a meltdown that can cost you your freedom or safety.

Building a Support System for Anger Control

Your friends, mentors, or family members can be part of your plan to keep anger in check. Let them know you are working on handling anger better. Ask them to gently tell you if they notice you getting wound up. If you trust them, you might even have a code word. When they say that word, you realize you are on the edge and need to calm down.

You can also meet people in anger management groups who share the same goal. Supporting each other can make the process easier. You learn from each other's mistakes and successes.

Turning Anger into Productive Action

In some cases, anger can motivate you. If you feel angry about certain injustices, you might channel that emotion into community service or honest activism. Instead of letting anger rot inside you, turn it into a drive to make positive changes in your neighborhood or in your own life.

For example, if you hate the fact that younger men in your area are turning to gangs, you might volunteer for a youth program to give them better options. This way, your anger becomes a fuel for something constructive rather than destructive.

Checking Your Thoughts

Anger often grows when we think certain thoughts, such as: "They are doing this on purpose," or "No one respects me." In reality, the other person might not be aiming to hurt you. Maybe they had a bad day or did not realize they were being rude. Learning to question your first assumption can cut down on anger.

Ask yourself: "Is there another explanation for what happened?" For example, if a friend did not call you back, maybe they got busy or lost their phone. Jumping to "He is ignoring me" can spark needless rage. By checking your thoughts, you keep anger from running wild.

Rewarding Yourself for Progress

As you learn to handle your anger better, reward yourself in small ways. It can be as simple as watching a favorite show when you handle a tough situation calmly. Or having a treat if you go a week without blowing up. You are training your mind to see that good behavior leads to good feelings. This might sound simple, but it can be very effective.

Over time, the satisfaction of being in control of your anger becomes its own reward. You will notice your body feels better when you are not tense all the time. Your relationships may improve. You might get more respect at work or among friends. These positive changes reinforce your new habits.

Conclusion of Chapter 4

Handling anger in a healthy way is not about never feeling mad. It is about recognizing when anger rises, understanding why it is there, and taking steps so it does not lead you down a dark path. Whether it is learning to breathe deeply, leaving the room, writing in a journal, or talking to a counselor, these methods can keep you in control.

After prison, you have enough challenges without letting anger destroy your chances at a better life. By being aware of your triggers, practicing new reactions, and finding ways to cool off, you show yourself and others that you can handle stress responsibly. In the long run, this can help you keep your freedom, your health, and your relationships intact.

Remember, anger can wreck or it can be turned into a force for personal improvement. The choice is in your hands. Each time you resist an outburst or apologize for a slip, you are shaping a better future. This does not mean you become a doormat. You can stand up for yourself without blowing up. That middle ground—staying calm but firm—is where true power lies.

Chapter 5: Finding a Stable Place to Live

When you get out of prison, one of the first hurdles you might face is finding a decent place to live. Without stable housing, it is harder to hold a job, care for your health, or focus on building better habits. This chapter offers a practical look at how to find housing, even when your record might limit your choices. You will learn about different housing options, what to expect in rental applications, ways to handle background checks, and tips on keeping your place once you have it.

---

1. Why Stable Housing Matters

A stable home is more than just a roof over your head. It is the foundation that supports all other parts of your life. If you do not have a reliable place to stay, you could end up couch-surfing or sleeping in places that are unsafe. That kind of life adds stress. When you do not feel safe, it is harder to keep a steady job or maintain your well-being.

Having your own place (or a safe shared place) also gives you privacy. It is where you can make plans for the future, manage your belongings, and rest without worrying about being kicked out the next morning. Many men overlook how big a difference it makes to come home each day to a spot that does not change.

---

2. Types of Housing Options

a) Transitional Housing or Halfway Houses

Some organizations offer short-term housing for people who have just left prison. These places often have rules, such as curfews or mandatory check-ins, but they can serve as a stepping stone. You might have a shared bedroom or dorm-like setup. The advantage is that staff there might help you connect with jobs, counseling, or other community resources. The downside is that space might be limited, and you often cannot stay for very long.

b) Renting a Room

If you cannot afford a full apartment, renting a room in someone's house or apartment might be a good option. You can find such listings online or posted on community bulletin boards. This can be cheaper than renting your own place. On the flip side, you have to share common areas (kitchen, living room, bathroom) with others. Be sure to get clear rules about rent, use of the kitchen, and any expectations about chores or visitors.

c) Living with Family

Some men move back in with their parents, siblings, or other relatives. This can help you save money and have a support system right away. However, it can also bring its own challenges, especially if relationships are tense. Make sure to talk about house rules and how you will contribute financially or help out. This might include cleaning, buying groceries, or paying some share of the bills. If you do not discuss these things, conflicts can arise.

d) Supportive Housing Programs

In some areas, nonprofit groups run supportive housing programs specifically for people with records. These programs might help with job training, counseling, and case management. You might have to follow certain conditions, such as attending support meetings or passing regular check-ins. The benefit is that you get more than just a place to sleep—you get help in rebuilding your life.

e) Renting an Apartment on Your Own

If you can afford it and pass the application requirements, renting your own unit gives you the most privacy and control. But it can also be the hardest route if you have a record, because landlords may do background checks. You also need the money for a security deposit, first month's rent, and possibly last month's rent. If you are on parole or probation, make sure your address is approved by your supervising officer.

---

3. Budgeting for Housing

Before you sign any rental agreement, you should figure out how much you can realistically afford. Most finance experts advise that housing should not be more than about 30% of your income. If you make $1,500 a month, try to keep your rent around $450 or less. That might not be easy in some areas, so you might need to share a place with roommates or look for a smaller unit.

If you have no job yet, try to get some form of income as soon as possible. This could be a part-time job, day labor, or a short-term work program. Use some of that income to start building up a little savings for your move-in costs. Even saving $20 a week can help with future deposits or emergency repairs.

---

4. Searching for Housing

a) Online Resources

Many landlords and people looking for roommates post listings on sites like Craigslist or other housing websites. You can filter by price range and location. Be ready to see many listings that do not mention anything about criminal records. You will likely have to address that issue during the application or interview phase.

b) Community Boards

Some towns have community bulletin boards in grocery stores, libraries, or laundromats. People post flyers for rooms or apartments for rent. This old-school approach might be helpful in smaller areas. You can also ask staff at community centers or your parole office if they know of any local leads.

c) Word of Mouth

Tell trusted friends, family members, or mentors that you are looking for a stable place. Sometimes, informal connections open doors that online searches do not. Maybe a friend of a friend has a basement for rent or needs a roommate. Still, be cautious. Always check the environment to make sure it is safe and not connected to any illegal activity.

---

5. Handling Background Checks

Many landlords run background checks to see if you have a record. Some might reject you immediately upon seeing a felony. Others might ask for an explanation. Be ready to talk about what happened and how you have changed. A few tips:

1. **Honesty**: Lying about your record can lead to eviction later if the landlord finds out. It is better to be upfront.

2. **Show Growth**: If you have completed a program in prison, or if you have letters of recommendation from counselors or employers, bring them. These documents can help show you are working hard to stay on track.
3. **Keep It Brief**: You do not have to share every detail of your crime. Be clear about the basics and focus on what you are doing now to move forward.

Some states or cities have "fair chance" housing laws that forbid landlords from rejecting you solely based on your record (unless it is related to certain serious crimes). Read up on the rules where you live, or ask a legal aid group for guidance.

---

6. Building References

A reference is someone who can speak up for you. Many rental applications ask for references to confirm that you will pay on time and keep the place in good shape. If you just got out of prison, you might not have a recent landlord reference. That is where other people can help:

- **Employer or Job Trainer**: If you are working or have completed a job-training program, ask the supervisor for a letter stating that you show up on time and work well with others.
- **Parole Officer or Counselor**: Some officers or counselors may be willing to vouch that you are following your conditions and making an honest effort to do well.
- **Volunteers or Mentors**: If you are involved in any reentry program or volunteering, those coordinators can sometimes give references about your reliability.

Have these references ready, typed up or in letter form, so you can hand them to landlords along with your application. It signals that you are prepared and serious.

---

7. Saving for Deposits and Move-In Costs

Moving into a new place typically requires a security deposit plus the first month's rent. Sometimes, landlords also want last month's rent upfront. If you do not have that kind of money, it can feel impossible. Here are a few ideas:

1. **Short-Term Jobs**: Seek day-labor gigs or part-time work to build up savings quickly.
2. **Assistance Programs**: Some charities or nonprofits offer small grants or loans to help with deposits if you meet their conditions.
3. **Ask Family**: If your relatives are willing and able, they might lend you the deposit if they see you are serious about building a stable life. Write down the loan terms so you can pay them back gradually.
4. **Shared Housing**: Splitting costs with a roommate can cut your part of the deposit in half or more.

The key is not to sign a lease unless you have a realistic plan to cover all move-in costs without leaving yourself penniless for food and transportation.

---

8. The Rental Application Process

When you fill out a rental application, you typically give personal information like your name, employment details, previous addresses, and references. The landlord may ask for a small fee to run a background and credit check. Some tips to stand out:

- **Complete the Form Fully**: Leaving blank spaces makes you look careless.
- **Offer Extra Documents**: Show pay stubs, reference letters, or any other proof of reliability.
- **Stay Polite and Respectful**: How you treat the landlord during your first meeting can make a big difference.

If you get rejected, ask politely if there was a specific reason (like the record or credit score). This helps you know what to improve next time. Some landlords might be open to suggestions like paying a slightly larger deposit or getting a co-signer if that makes them more comfortable.

---

9. Considering Roommates or Housemates

Sharing a place can save you money, but you have to be careful about who you choose. If you live with someone involved in illegal activity, that could pull you back into trouble. Also, living with friends might seem nice at first, but if they are irresponsible with rent or disrespectful of your privacy, it can ruin the friendship and threaten your housing stability.

Before you agree to live with someone, have a direct talk about rent splitting, cleaning duties, visitors, and what happens if someone cannot pay. Having these details in writing can prevent arguments later.

---

10. Basic Housekeeping Skills

Some men have never lived on their own before or had to keep a space tidy. But landlords and neighbors do not want someone who will trash the place. Keep these points in mind:

- **Cleaning Schedule**: Do a quick daily cleanup—wash dishes after meals, wipe counters, sweep if needed. Then plan a bigger cleaning once a week (vacuuming, scrubbing the bathroom, etc.).
- **Trash Removal**: Put trash out on time to avoid odors or pests.
- **Repairs**: If something breaks, tell the landlord promptly. Do not hide problems because they can get worse and cost more.
- **Respect Neighbors**: Keep noise levels reasonable, especially late at night.

Keeping your place tidy and in good condition builds trust with the landlord and neighbors. That trust can come in handy if you need a positive reference later or an extension on rent due to an emergency.

---

11. Dealing with Rules and Neighbors

If you are on probation or parole, you might have extra rules about who can visit or whether you can have alcohol in the home. Make sure you follow these conditions so you do not jeopardize your freedom. You might also face building rules about quiet hours, pets, or parking. Break these rules too often, and you risk eviction.

Neighbors can be a source of stress if they complain about noise or suspect you of something because of your record. Try to keep communication open. If someone has a concern, listen calmly. If they are rude or make false claims, involve your landlord only if needed, and remain polite. Avoid letting minor conflicts blow up into a bigger problem. By showing respect and staying calm, you can reduce friction.

---

12. Staying Safe in Your New Home

After living in prison, you might feel the need to be on guard. One way to feel more secure is to make sure your doors and windows lock properly. If you have any issues with locks, ask the landlord to fix them. You can also get inexpensive battery-powered alarms or doorstop alarms for extra peace of mind.

Be aware of your surroundings. If you see suspicious activity near your home, you can quietly keep track and share it with the landlord or call a non-emergency police line (if needed). But also be cautious about who you let inside. Do not invite people you barely know into your room or apartment. Remember, you can lose your lease if your guests cause damage or do anything illegal.

---

13. Overcoming Rejections

You might face several "no" answers before you find a landlord or housing program that will accept you. It can be discouraging, but it is not the end. Treat each rejection as part of the process. There are more potential rentals out there. Here are some actions you can take after a rejection:

- **Review Your Approach**: Was your application fully filled out? Were you upfront about your record? Could you improve your references or presentation next time?
- **Seek Programs That Help**: There may be housing-focused nonprofits that can assist with deposits, negotiations, or legal advice.
- **Stay Positive**: The more you learn from each rejection, the better you can handle the next application.

Remember, you only need one "yes" to make progress. Keep applying until you find a match.

---

14. Planning for Long-Term Housing Security

Once you find a stable place, you might still want to move to a better neighborhood or larger unit in the future. That is completely fine. Use your current spot as a stepping stone. In the meantime:

- **Pay Rent on Time**: Late payments can lead to eviction. If you ever have money troubles, communicate with the landlord beforehand.
- **Build Good Tenant History**: Follow the lease rules, keep the place clean, and be friendly with neighbors. Over time, you will have a record as a responsible tenant.
- **Improve Your Finances**: Work on steady income, build savings, and maybe improve your credit score if that is an option. This will open doors to better housing later on.

---

15. Special Tip: Look for "Second Chance" Landlords

Some landlords specialize in renting to people who have records. They might have a more lenient view on background checks, focusing instead on whether you can pay rent and stay out of trouble. These landlords might be found through reentry programs, local community centers, or word of mouth. They may still have requirements, such as no drug use on the property or proof of employment, but they are often more open to giving you a shot than mainstream landlords.

---

16. Avoiding Old Traps

Be cautious if old friends who are still in crime offer you a place to crash. Sure, it may solve your housing issue for a while, but it can also drag you back into risky behavior. The same goes for areas or buildings known for heavy drug use or illegal activities. If your goal is to stay out of trouble, your environment matters. Try to find a living arrangement that helps you move forward, not pull you back.

---

17. Using a Housing Advocate (If Available)

Some cities have advocates who help people with records navigate the housing process. These advocates can speak on your behalf to landlords, help with paperwork, or direct you to programs you did not know about. If you find one, use their expertise. They might also connect you with legal aid if a landlord discriminates against you in violation of local laws.

---

18. Handling Legal Lease Documents

When you are ready to sign a lease, read it carefully. Many people sign without understanding the terms. Look for details on:

- **Length of Lease**: Is it month-to-month or for a full year?
- **Rent Amount and Due Date**: How much you owe and when is it due?
- **Security Deposit**: How much and under what conditions can you get it back?
- **Rules**: Are there limits on visitors, overnight guests, noise, or storage?
- **Penalties**: What happens if you pay late? What about damages?

If anything is unclear, ask questions before you sign. Once you sign, you are legally bound. Keep a copy of the lease for your records. If you do not own a printer, you can take clear pictures of it on your phone.

---

19. The Day You Move In

Moving day can be exciting and stressful. Do a quick walk-through with the landlord. Note any existing damage (holes, stains, broken fixtures) and take pictures. Share these with the landlord so you are not blamed for them later. If something is in bad shape, ask when it will be fixed. Organize your belongings, keep the place tidy from day one, and introduce yourself politely to neighbors if you see them in passing.

---

20. Conclusion of Chapter 5

Finding stable housing after prison might feel like a huge obstacle, but it is a problem you can tackle step by step. You can start with short-term options like transitional housing, then move on to renting a room or an apartment as you build your finances and references. Do not give up if you hear "no" many times. Each search teaches you something new.

Stable housing is the cornerstone for everything else—work, relationships, personal growth. By having a safe and reliable place to call home, you lay the groundwork for a more secure life. Show landlords you are responsible, stay on top of your bills, and keep the property in good shape. Over time, you build a positive rental history, making it easier to find housing in the future.

Chapter 6: Creating Support Through Friends and Groups

Life after prison can feel lonely, especially if you lost contact with people while you were locked up. It helps to have others around you who can understand your struggles, offer practical help, and share ideas. This chapter looks at how to build or rebuild a support network, from reconnecting with old friends to finding new groups that can guide you.

---

1. Why a Support Network Matters

No one succeeds alone. After prison, you might face tough times—rejections, stress, regret, money problems, and more. Friends, family, mentors, or community groups can step in to offer emotional backing, job leads, or a shoulder to lean on. A strong support network can make the difference between moving ahead or sliding back into old habits.

You are not "weak" for leaning on others. In fact, knowing when to seek help is a sign of strength. A good support system does not do all the work for you, but it keeps you motivated and reduces the feeling that you are all by yourself.

---

2. Types of Support

a) Emotional Support

These are people who will listen to your problems without judging. They might not always have a solution, but just having someone care about how you feel can ease stress. Emotional supporters can be close friends, siblings, or even folks you meet in group sessions.

b) Practical Support

Practical supporters offer hands-on help. That could mean driving you to a job interview, helping you learn to write a resume, or teaching you a skill. Mentors, community volunteers, and some family members can give this kind of support. It is helpful to have at least one person in your life who can show you practical ways to move forward.

c) Professional Support

Professional supporters include counselors, therapists, parole officers, case workers, and others with specific roles. They are there to guide you in certain areas like mental health, legal issues, or job placement. They might not be your buddies, but their expertise can help you solve serious problems.

---

3. Reconnecting with Old Friends

If you had friends who stayed out of trouble and are leading stable lives, you might try reaching out to them. A simple phone call or message can break the ice. Be honest about your situation and ask if they are open to hanging out or talking. Some might have moved on, or they might feel uncertain about you. That is normal. But a few might be glad to hear from you.

Keep in mind that if old friends are still involved in crime or dangerous habits, it might not be healthy to reconnect too closely. You can wish them well without getting pulled back into risky behavior. Choose friends who add something good to your life rather than drag you down.

---

4. Building New Friendships

Sometimes, you have to form new social ties. This can be hard if you are shy or if you are used to prison life where trust is not freely given. A few ways to meet new people:

1. **Community Events**: Look for free local gatherings at libraries, cultural centers, or parks.
2. **Interest-Based Groups**: If you like sports, join a local team or league. If you enjoy art or music, see if there is a casual group you can attend. You bond faster when you share a common interest.
3. **Volunteer Work**: Helping out at a nonprofit or food bank is a chance to do good and meet people who also want to help.
4. **Support Groups**: There are specific groups for men reentering society, substance recovery groups, or faith-based fellowships.

Take it slow. You do not have to share your entire past right away. But as you feel comfortable, open up about your goals and what you are trying to achieve. That honesty can form deeper connections.

---

5. Being Selective About Your Circle

Not everyone who smiles at you is a true ally. Some might see your past as a weakness they can exploit. Others might think you are an easy target for illegal plans. Be mindful of who you let into your inner circle.

- **Watch Their Actions**: Do they keep their word? Do they treat others with respect? Or do they lie and manipulate?
- **Notice Their Values**: Are they trying to do well in life, or do they shrug off rules and push you toward risky choices?
- **See How They React to Your Boundaries**: Good friends respect your limits. They do not push you to break your parole or skip your responsibilities.

Cutting ties with people who encourage bad behavior might feel lonely at first, but it is often necessary to stay out of prison. A smaller circle of genuine friends is better than a large group of shady connections.

---

6. Group Support Sessions

a) Reentry Support Groups

These groups bring together people who have been in prison and are now trying to live well. They often share tips about jobs, housing, and coping with shame or stress. Being in a group like this can make you realize you are not alone. You can learn from others' successes and failures.

b) Faith-Based Groups

Churches, mosques, temples, or other faith groups sometimes have special meetings or ministries for men coming out of prison. You do not have to be deeply religious to attend. These gatherings might offer prayer, moral support, or community service. They can also introduce you to mentors who have overcome similar pasts.

c) Therapy or Counseling Groups

Some mental health clinics offer group therapy sessions for anger problems, sadness, or addiction. In these groups, you get professional guidance while also hearing from people in similar situations. You practice new ways of thinking and behaving. This can be more structured than casual support groups, but it can also be very effective if you need deeper help.

---

7. Mentors and Role Models

A mentor is someone with more experience who is willing to guide you. This might be a neighbor who has stayed on the right path, a small-business owner who wants to hire men with records, or a program coordinator who helps with reentry services. A mentor is not just a friend. They give direct advice, share life lessons, and sometimes hold you accountable.

If you find a potential mentor, be clear about what you are hoping for. Maybe you want job search tips, or you need guidance on staying away from criminal crowds. Be respectful of their time. If they set up a meeting, show up on time. If they give you a suggestion, at least consider it seriously. Mentors often enjoy helping someone who is truly trying.

---

8. Online Communities

In the modern world, not all support is face-to-face. You might find online groups or forums for people who have been in prison. These groups can share stories, advice, and resources. While the internet can be helpful, remember not to trust everyone you meet online. Some people pose as friends but have hidden motives. Keep personal details (like exact address or banking info) private until you really know who you are talking to.

If you join social media groups, look for those with a track record of serious discussions and respectful behavior. Avoid groups where people only complain or encourage illegal activities. That will not help you move forward.

9. Contributing to Your Network

Friendship and group support are not just about receiving help. They are also about giving back. When you offer help to others in your circle, you strengthen those ties. This does not mean giving money you do not have. It can be small things like:

- Sharing a job lead you found.
- Helping someone study for a driving test or a GED.
- Listening when a friend is stressed.
- Encouraging them to avoid old traps.

When you give to others, you prove to yourself and them that you have something valuable to offer. This boosts your confidence and bonds the group more closely.

---

10. Handling Conflicts in Friendships

No friendship is perfect. Sometimes you will clash with a friend or group member. Maybe you disagree on how to handle a certain situation or you feel they are not respecting your time. Here are some basic conflict-resolution tips:

1. **Stay Calm**: Do not let anger take over. Cool down before addressing the issue.
2. **Use Respectful Language**: Avoid name-calling or accusations. Instead, focus on the behavior or situation that bothered you.
3. **Listen**: Hear their side without interrupting. Maybe there is a misunderstanding.
4. **Look for Solutions**: Figure out what each person needs. Is there a compromise or a way to meet in the middle?
5. **Know When to Walk Away**: If the conflict becomes toxic or the person refuses to respect your boundaries, it might be time to keep your distance.

Resolving conflicts in a mature way is a skill that will help you in jobs, relationships, and everyday life.

---

11. Family Support

Your family can be part of your support network if they are reliable and caring. However, some family dynamics are complicated. You might have family members who blame you for past burdens, or who are themselves caught up in harmful behavior. If you have a supportive family, that is great—cherish those ties and show them you appreciate their help.

If your family situation is toxic, you might need to keep contact limited while you work on your stability. It is a tough choice, but your freedom and well-being come first. Over time, you can try to rebuild family bonds if both sides are willing to do the work.

---

12. Peer Accountability Partnerships

A peer accountability partnership is when two or more people agree to keep each other on track. For example, if you and a friend both want to avoid certain bad habits, you can check in with each other daily or weekly. You can ask, "How are you doing with your goals? Did you slip up?" If one of you is struggling, the other can offer reminders or tips.

This works best when both parties are serious about self-improvement. It gives you someone who understands your situation and can hold you responsible for your actions. It is like having a teammate who wants you to succeed, and you want them to succeed too.

---

13. Asking for Help When You Need It

Many men are taught to solve everything on their own and never ask for help. This mindset can lead to isolation. Real strength includes knowing when to reach out. If you are facing a crisis—such as homelessness, job loss, or legal trouble—do not suffer alone. Tell a friend, call a helpline, or visit a community center. Even if they cannot fix the situation, they might point you to resources or people who can.

Asking for help does not mean you are failing. It means you recognize you are at your limit and need backup. This is something even the strongest men do at times.

14. Steering Clear of Harmful Influences

Being out of prison does not mean everyone around you will want you to do the right thing. Some folks might try to pull you back into illegal activities. Others might tempt you to abuse substances. Part of building a good support network is guarding it against negative influences.

- **Say "No" Clearly**: If someone invites you to a place or activity that risks your parole or your safety, do not beat around the bush. Say you cannot go and explain you are focused on building a better life.
- **Do Not Let Guilt Pressure You**: Some might say you are "too good" for them now, or you have changed. That is okay. You do not owe them your future freedom.
- **Keep Your Goals in Mind**: Whenever you feel drawn to old ways, remind yourself why you are staying on this path—maybe for your children, your own peace of mind, or to avoid going back to a jail cell.

---

15. Making the Most of Organized Programs

Many organizations exist to help those returning from prison. These groups might have classes on job readiness, free legal clinics, or even group outings to practice social skills in a safe setting. Check if your parole office or local nonprofits have such programs. Attending regularly helps you meet other folks in the same boat, and you might find a mentor or friend.

These programs can also keep you accountable since they often track attendance. Staying active shows that you are serious about starting a new chapter and can help when you need recommendations for housing or employment.

---

16. Being a Positive Influence

Over time, as you get more stable, you can become a positive influence for others coming out of prison. You do not need a fancy title to do this. Maybe you share tips with a younger man about how to find housing. Maybe you encourage someone to keep going to group sessions. When you lift others up, you reinforce your own progress. It is a reminder of how far you have come and why you want to stay on the right side.

17. Avoiding the Lone-Wolf Trap

A common mistake is trying to handle every challenge alone. You might think, "I will do it all myself so no one can let me down." But isolation can lead to depression, relapse into bad habits, and lack of progress. Strong individuals still need allies. A team can achieve more than a single person, especially when the road is full of obstacles like background checks, social stigma, or personal doubts.

When you feel the urge to push everyone away, do the opposite. Reach out to at least one trusted contact or attend a support meeting. Just being around people who understand can lift your mood and remind you that you do not have to do everything on your own.

---

18. Keeping Up Long-Term Support

Building support is not a one-time event. You do not just join a group, make a friend, or see a counselor once and call it done. These connections need regular upkeep. That might mean:

- Checking in with friends weekly to ask how they are doing.
- Staying consistent in group meetings, not just dropping by when you feel like it.
- Being open about changes in your life so people can help you if things get tough.

Long-term support networks can last for years. Over time, you might see your friends settle down, get better jobs, or even start families. You will be growing along with them, sharing each other's triumphs and helping through hard times.

---

19. Tips for Expanding Your Network Safely

- **Attend Local Workshops**: If you hear about a free workshop on budgeting or computer skills, go. You might learn something new and meet people in similar situations.
- **Look into Sports or Fitness Groups**: Physical activity is healthy, and team sports or group fitness classes can help you connect with others.

- **Check Out Community Centers**: These places often host events, classes, or general hangouts. Strike up a conversation with someone there.
- **Speak Up Politely**: If you meet someone interesting, do not be afraid to introduce yourself. You can say, "I am looking to learn more about this program. Can you tell me how you got involved?" Simple questions can spark a friendship.

---

20. Conclusion of Chapter 6

Creating a support system after prison is a major part of building a life that keeps you out of trouble and moving in a better direction. People around you can offer different kinds of help—emotional, practical, and professional. Whether you reconnect with old friends, find new ones, or join groups designed to help you, the main point is that you do not have to carry every burden alone.

Be selective in who you trust. Choose those who respect your boundaries and push you toward good things, not back into crime. When conflicts arise, handle them with maturity. Give back to your circle by offering help when you can. Over time, you will see that a solid support network can keep you motivated, teach you new skills, and help you recover after missteps.

You might have days when you feel like no one understands. That is when group meetings, mentors, or a single good friend can make a huge difference. Remember, strong support does not mean you are reliant on others for everything. It means you have people who believe in your ability to succeed. Use their belief to strengthen your own, and you will be far less likely to return to the old ways that led to prison.

Chapter 7: Getting a Job and Building Work Skills

A stable job is one of the biggest stepping stones toward a solid life after prison. Earning a steady paycheck helps you pay rent, buy food, and reduce stress about basic needs. It also gives you a sense of direction each day. But finding employment with a record can be tough. This chapter looks at practical ways to look for job openings, handle interviews, improve your skills, and hold onto the job once you have it.

---

1. Why Work Matters

Having a job is not just about money. It provides structure, new contacts, and a sense of pride. When you wake up each day knowing you have a task to do, it often keeps your mind from drifting to bad habits. A job can also help you prove to yourself (and to others) that you can stick with something and succeed, regardless of your past.

Furthermore, many employers or landlords want to see proof of reliable income before considering you. When you can show a steady work history, it opens doors for housing, loans, and more. In short, a solid job can greatly reduce the risk of returning to prison because it gives you fewer reasons to engage in illegal ways to make money.

---

2. Dealing with the Record Issue

One of the hardest parts of finding work after prison is knowing how to address your record. Some job applications still ask if you have been convicted of a crime. Others do not ask but will run a background check. While it can be frustrating, you can use these strategies:

1. **Honesty**: If asked, do not lie about your record. Getting caught in a lie can be worse than the record itself, because it shows dishonesty.
2. **Keep It Short**: When explaining your record, stick to the basics: what the charge was, how long you served, and that you are now focused on doing better.
3. **Highlight Growth**: Talk about classes, certifications, or programs you did while inside. Show that you used your time constructively.

4. **Use References**: If you have a mentor, counselor, or former boss (from a prison job program or a reentry program) willing to speak for you, mention them. Positive references can ease concerns about hiring someone with a record.

Some cities or states have "ban the box" rules that limit what an employer can ask about your record during the early phases of hiring. If you live in such an area, you might get a fairer chance to show your skills before background questions come up. Look up local laws or ask a reentry agency for details.

---

3. Types of Jobs to Consider

a) Entry-Level Positions

These are roles that do not require special training or a long work history. Examples include warehouse work, fast food, cleaning, landscaping, construction labor, and retail stocking. Pay might be low at first, but they can help you build a stable work record.

b) Trades and Vocational Work

If you have skills in carpentry, welding, electrical work, plumbing, or other trades, you might find decent-paying jobs. Some employers in these fields are more willing to hire people with records, especially if there is a labor shortage. If you do not have these skills yet, consider enrolling in a training program. Many community colleges and nonprofits offer short courses.

c) Temp Agencies

Temporary staffing agencies match workers with companies that need short-term help. You might be placed in different roles, like assembly lines, moving jobs, or basic office tasks. While temp work is not always steady, it can help you gain experience and show a potential employer that you are reliable. Sometimes, a temp job can turn into a full-time position if you perform well.

d) Food Industry

Restaurants, catering businesses, and food production plants often need staff for dishwashing, prep work, or line cooking. If you enjoy food service and can handle fast-paced environments, you might find opportunities here. Some places will hire you even with a record, as they care more about your punctuality and willingness to learn.

e) Self-Employment or Freelancing

If you have a skill like auto repair, cleaning, painting, cutting hair, or any other service, you can try working for yourself. You can start small—maybe fix cars in your neighborhood or offer lawn-care services. This avoids some of the background check issues. But you must be ready for the business side of things: setting fair prices, advertising, and managing your income. Over time, you can build a customer base and make it a steady source of money.

---

4. Searching for Job Leads

a) Online Job Boards

Websites like Indeed, CareerBuilder, or other local job boards list thousands of openings. You can filter by location, part-time or full-time, and see what matches your skill level. Make sure you have a simple resume ready to upload, or fill out the online forms carefully.

b) Community Centers and Nonprofits

Some organizations focus on helping people with records find work. They might have job listings, training programs, or direct links to employers who are open to hiring. They can also help with resume writing and interview prep. Local community centers, churches, or reentry programs are often good places to ask for leads.

c) Networking

Sometimes, the best way to find a job is through people you already know—friends, family, neighbors, or mentors. Let them know you are looking for work. If you have a clean and honest record with them (meaning they trust you now), they might introduce you to someone who is hiring. Be clear about what kind of jobs you are open to and whether you can work different shifts.

d) Career Fairs

Some cities hold career fairs, often at convention centers or community colleges, where multiple employers set up booths. You can meet hiring managers face-to-face and hand them your resume. It is a chance to make a quick, positive impression, which might help them overlook any record concerns. Dress neatly, be polite, and show interest in the company.

---

5. Resume Basics

A resume is a short document that summarizes your work experience, skills, and education. If you have gaps in your history due to prison time, you can mention "personal leave" or be ready to discuss it briefly if asked. Here are some resume tips:

- **Contact Info**: Your name, phone number, and email address at the top.
- **Objective Statement**: A brief line about the job you want or the skills you bring.
- **Work Experience**: List any relevant work, even if it was in prison (kitchen work, laundry, maintenance, etc.). Explain your duties in a professional way (e.g., "Managed inventory, followed safety rules, supervised cleaning tasks").
- **Education and Training**: List high school, GED, vocational certifications, or any other courses you completed.
- **Skills**: Highlight both soft skills (teamwork, communication) and hard skills (forklift operation, basic welding, etc.).
- **References**: Mention "Available upon request" unless the employer specifically asks for them up front.

If your resume is very short, consider a "skills-based" layout. Focus on what you can do well rather than a strict timeline of jobs. This can be helpful if your job gaps are large.

---

6. Preparing for Interviews

An interview is your chance to show an employer who you are beyond the resume. Even if you feel nervous, remember that an interview is just a conversation. Some pointers:

1. **Dress Appropriately**: Clean, well-fitting clothes. You do not need a fancy suit unless the job is in a corporate setting. For many entry-level or labor jobs, a neat shirt and pants will do.

2. **Arrive Early**: Plan to get there 10–15 minutes before the interview time. Being late can kill your chances immediately.
3. **Have Good Posture**: Stand and sit up straight. Offer a firm handshake if that is normal in your region. Make eye contact but do not stare.
4. **Answer Questions Directly**: Speak clearly. If they ask about your strengths, mention skills or traits that relate to the job (e.g., reliable, good with hands, fast learner).
5. **Handle the Record Topic**: If it comes up, address it calmly. Explain that you made mistakes in the past but have worked to change. Point out anything positive you achieved since then.
6. **Ask Questions**: Show interest in the company. You might ask, "What does a typical day look like in this role?" or "What qualities do you value most in your employees?"

If you feel very anxious, practice with a friend or mentor. Role-play the interview. They can give feedback on your answers and body language.

---

7. Overcoming Common Barriers

You might face problems such as:

- **Lack of Transportation**: If you do not have a car, plan for public transport or ask a friend in advance for a ride. Arriving late because you do not have a ride is an avoidable mistake.
- **Limited Work Clothes**: If you only have one decent outfit, wash and iron it before interviews. Some nonprofits give free or low-cost work attire to job seekers who need it.
- **Negative Employer Attitudes**: Some bosses will reject you outright if they see a record. Do not take it personally. Focus on those who are open to giving you a chance.

If you get turned down for a job, try to learn something from that experience. Perhaps you can improve your interview skills or target different industries. Rejection is normal for any job seeker. Keep at it.

8. On-the-Job Behavior and Retention

Once you get hired, the next challenge is keeping the job and building a good reputation. Here are key points:

1. **Reliability**: Show up on time every day. If you are sick or have an emergency, call early and let them know. Do not just vanish without explanation.
2. **Work Ethic**: Do your tasks thoroughly. If you finish, ask if there is more you can do. Employers appreciate workers who show initiative.
3. **Respect the Chain of Command**: Follow instructions from your supervisor. If you have a disagreement, handle it politely or ask for a private talk rather than losing your temper on the spot.
4. **Learn New Skills**: Show interest in different tasks around the workplace. You might get trained on more machines or tasks, which can lead to raises or promotions.
5. **Avoid Gossip**: Stay clear of workplace drama. Keep conversations respectful and avoid negative talk about coworkers or the boss.
6. **Document Everything**: If you complete a job-related course or get any positive feedback, save it. This can help you advance to better positions later.

---

9. Handling Stress at Work

Jobs can be stressful, especially if you have been away from normal work life for a while. If a boss or customer is rude, do not snap. Use anger control techniques (see Chapter 4) and remember that losing your cool can cost you your job. After a tough day, find healthy outlets like exercise, talking to a friend, or a hobby.

Also, watch out for burnout. Working long hours or multiple jobs to make ends meet can drain you. Try to maintain a balance: rest when you can, eat properly, and keep up small social connections. A stable job is good, but not if it leads to exhaustion that harms your health or relationships.

---

10. Climbing the Ladder

You do not have to stay in an entry-level job forever. Once you have a foot in the door, aim to move up. Ask your supervisor about any training or advancement paths. Offer to learn new roles. If you prove yourself capable, many employers prefer to promote from within, because training an existing employee can be easier than hiring a new one.

Even if the company does not offer promotions, the skills you gain can help you apply for better jobs elsewhere. Every new piece of experience—operating a forklift, handling cash, dealing with customers, writing reports—expands your resume and your opportunities.

---

11. Education and Skills Improvement

A job might pay the bills now, but improving your skills can lead to better-paying work. You can:

- **Get a GED**: If you did not finish high school, this certificate can open more doors. Many adult education centers offer free classes.
- **Attend Vocational or Trade School**: Look for part-time programs in welding, electrical, plumbing, automotive repair, HVAC, or culinary arts. Skilled trades often pay well and have decent demand.
- **Learn Computer Basics**: Even simple office or warehouse jobs often require basic computer use (email, data entry). Libraries or community centers sometimes have free classes.
- **Seek Apprenticeships**: Some unions or trade groups have paid programs where you learn a skill on the job while also taking related classes. You earn while you learn, although these can be competitive to get into.

Balancing work and classes can be tiring, but it is an investment in your future. Each new skill reduces the risk of unemployment and raises your earning potential.

---

12. Networking for Better Opportunities

Once you are working, keep building connections. Talk politely with coworkers, attend company events (if you feel comfortable), and ask about any local trade groups. If you show a professional attitude, some folks might recommend you for other positions, or let you know when their friend's business is hiring.

Always be respectful, but do not be afraid to let people know your goals. For example, if you dream of becoming a supervisor or starting your own small business, share that ambition with trusted contacts. People might point you to resources or introduce you to someone who can help.

---

13. Side Gigs and Extra Income

If your main job does not pay enough to cover all your expenses, you might consider a side gig. This could be:

- Driving for ride-share companies (if allowed in your area with your record).
- Doing yard work or handyman jobs on weekends.
- Cleaning offices after hours.
- Selling simple crafts or repaired goods online.

These extra efforts can help you build savings, pay off debts, or cover training fees for a better career. However, be mindful of burnout. You do not want to push yourself so hard that your health or your main job performance suffers.

---

14. Dealing with Discrimination or Setbacks

You might run into people who stereotype anyone with a record as untrustworthy. Or an employer might give you the worst tasks simply because they think you have no other option. If you feel unfairly targeted, document everything—dates, times, what was said. If it crosses the line into illegal discrimination (check local laws), you might seek legal advice or talk to a worker's rights group.

However, try to address minor issues professionally before jumping to legal action. Sometimes a calm chat with a supervisor can settle things. Show that you want to solve problems, not cause trouble.

Setbacks may also happen if you slip up at work, miss a shift, or struggle with the rules. Rather than quitting, own up to your mistakes and see if there is a way to fix the situation. Many managers appreciate honesty and might give you another chance if you show genuine effort.

15. Maintaining a Good Record on the Job

Building a positive track record is like creating your future resume in real time. Each month you stay employed without issues, your credibility grows. Keep an eye on:

- **Punctuality**: Be on time consistently.
- **Teamwork**: Cooperate with others, share credit, and help out when needed.
- **Quality Work**: Do tasks with care so they do not have to be redone.
- **Good Attitude**: Approach problems with a solution mindset instead of constant complaints.

If you do all these things, you can later ask your supervisor for a reference letter or to be listed as a reference. A positive review from a current or recent employer can outweigh much of the doubt some people may have about your record.

16. Balancing Parole or Probation with Work

If you are on supervised release, you might have to meet a parole or probation officer regularly. Sometimes you have classes or mandatory programs to attend. This can clash with your job schedule. The best approach is honesty:

- **Tell Your Employer**: You do not have to give all the details, but let them know you have mandatory appointments. Try to arrange them outside peak work hours if possible.
- **Plan Ahead**: Schedule meetings or check-ins in a way that causes minimal disruption to your shifts. Give your boss as much notice as you can for any necessary time off.
- **Stay in Communication**: Keep your officer updated on your job status and schedule. If your job requires you to travel or work different hours, make sure your supervising officer approves, if needed.

Skipping parole or probation requirements to keep your job can backfire. It might land you back in prison if you violate conditions. Try to coordinate so you can do both safely.

17. Building Confidence on the Job

Starting work after prison might feel scary. You may wonder if others look down on you or if you can keep up. Confidence grows with action. Each day you arrive on time and do your tasks, you prove to yourself you can succeed. If you make a mistake, own it, fix it, and learn from it. Over time, you will see that you have what it takes to hold a job and advance in your position.

Do not let every small error send you into a panic. Everyone slips up sometimes. Most bosses do not fire workers for a single mistake, as long as the worker stays honest and tries to improve. Believe in your ability to adapt and grow.

18. When to Look for a New Job

If your current job is low-paying or does not give enough hours, you might want to move on once you have gained some experience. Look for openings that pay better or offer more growth. But do not quit your current role before you have something else lined up (unless the situation is truly toxic or unsafe). Being unemployed can lead to financial stress that can push you toward poor choices.

By the time you are ready to look for a new job, you will have a work history and possibly references to back you up. That puts you in a stronger position than when you first got out of prison.

19. Handling Self-Doubt

Men who have been to prison often worry about whether they can compete in the workforce. You might fear rejection or wonder if all your efforts are a waste. Recognize that many people—record or not—face work challenges. The key is persistence. Each time you fill out an application, go to an interview, or learn a new skill, you are building your future.

If self-doubt grows overwhelming, talk to a counselor, support group, or a trusted friend. Remind yourself why you need this job: to stay free, to support your family, or to meet personal goals. Stay focused on what you can control—your behavior, your attitude, your willingness to learn.

20. Conclusion of Chapter 7

Getting a job after prison is a big step. It can be frustrating, especially when some employers reject you because of your record. But with persistence and planning, you can find a position that allows you to earn money, gain new skills, and build a better life.

Start by considering what kind of work you can do right now, then look for ways to improve your skills or education for better jobs down the road. Build a clear, honest resume and practice interview skills. Use local resources, family connections, and online tools to find openings. Be ready to address your record, but do not let it define you. Show employers that you are reliable, eager to learn, and prepared to move in a new direction.

Once you are hired, focus on being a dependable worker who respects the rules and strives to grow. Over time, that builds a solid job history that can help you move up in your field or switch to a better-paying role. You might even discover new talents you did not know you had. A steady job is not the only key to a better life, but it is one of the strongest pillars you can rely on as you continue building your future outside prison walls.

Chapter 8: Building Better Daily Routines

Routines might sound boring, but they can be the backbone of a stable life. A routine is simply a pattern of actions that you repeat every day or week. When you have been in prison, your schedule was often controlled by others—when to wake up, eat, exercise, or go to bed. After getting out, it is up to you to create your own structure. This can feel freeing but also confusing. This chapter examines how to build daily routines that keep you on track, reduce stress, and help you manage your time well.

---

1. Why Routines Matter

A daily routine does more than organize your day. It lowers the mental strain of deciding what to do next. When you know that you wake up at 6:00 a.m., shower, eat breakfast, and then head out, you avoid wasting time or falling back asleep. Routines can also help you reach long-term goals. Small repeated actions, like practicing a skill for 30 minutes each day, lead to big improvements over weeks and months.

Routines also give life a sense of predictability, which can be comforting after the unstable environment of prison. When you know what to expect from your day, you are less likely to feel lost or bored. Boredom can be dangerous because it sometimes pushes men toward old, harmful habits just to feel busy or alive.

---

2. Starting with the Morning

How you begin the day often sets the tone for the rest of it. A good morning routine might include:

1. **Fixed Wake-Up Time**: Aim for the same time each day. Use an alarm if needed.
2. **Quick Wash or Shower**: Wake yourself up, feel clean.
3. **Healthy Breakfast**: It can be something simple—oatmeal, eggs, or yogurt. If you do not have much time, prepare something the night before.
4. **Brief Planning**: Look at your schedule or to-do list for the day. Mentally note any key tasks.

5. **Positive Habit** (If time allows): This could be a short walk, simple stretching, or reading for ten minutes.

This morning pattern takes some discipline, but once it is locked in, you will start your day feeling organized. Some men say they never had a morning routine before prison, and that was part of the chaos that led them astray. By adding structure, you claim control over your life.

---

3. Planning Your Day

Try not to drift aimlessly. Write down or store on your phone a simple daily plan. This does not have to be fancy. It could look like:

- 7:00 a.m.: Breakfast and shower.
- 8:00 a.m.: Leave for work or job hunting.
- 12:00 p.m.: Lunch break.
- 1:00 p.m.: Resume work, training, or job search tasks.
- 5:00 p.m.: Return home, cook dinner.
- 6:30 p.m.: Check on personal errands, family time, or friend time.
- 8:00 p.m.: Light exercise or reading.
- 10:00 p.m.: Bedtime routine (shower, set clothes for tomorrow, etc.).

Adjust times based on your life. The key is to have a general framework so you know what should be happening at each part of the day. Some men find it helpful to use a planner or phone calendar with reminders. This is especially useful if you have parole meetings, counseling sessions, or other appointments. Missing these can cause big problems.

---

4. Balancing Work, Family, and Personal Needs

If you have a job, that likely takes a big chunk of your day. Add in travel time, and you might feel you have no hours left for yourself. Still, try to carve out time for personal needs (health, exercise, relaxation) and family or social relationships. For example:

- **Work Schedule**: 8 hours of the day (plus any commute).
- **Family Time**: A half hour to sit and talk, help with homework, or share a meal.

- **Personal Time**: Could be 15–30 minutes for reading, stretching, or just quiet reflection.
- **Errands**: Grocery shopping, paying bills, laundry.
- **Sleep**: At least 7 hours.

Yes, it can be tight. But planning each slot can keep you from feeling out of control. Even a short 10-minute chat with a loved one each day can keep you connected. Small efforts repeated often build healthy bonds.

---

5. Using Tools to Stay Organized

- **Calendars**: Physical calendars on your wall or digital ones on your phone can show you upcoming events at a glance.
- **To-Do Lists**: Write down the tasks you must do today. Check them off as you finish. This small action can give you a sense of achievement.
- **Alarms/Reminders**: If you need to pick up a prescription at 3:00 p.m., set an alert on your phone 15 minutes before. This helps you avoid forgetting important tasks.
- **Apps**: There are free apps that help with habit tracking, budgeting, and even meal planning. If you are comfortable with technology, these can be handy.

The main point is to reduce the burden on your memory. Life outside prison can have many moving parts. By writing things down or using digital reminders, you free your mind to focus on the tasks themselves rather than juggling dates and times.

---

6. Creating Positive Habits

A habit is something you do so often that it becomes nearly automatic. Building positive habits makes your routine smoother. Here are a few examples of helpful habits:

- **Daily Cleanup**: Spend 10 minutes picking up trash, washing dishes, or organizing. This keeps your living space tidy without big weekend clean-ups.
- **Budget Check**: Look at your budget weekly (or daily if needed) to track spending.

- **Skill Practice**: If you want to learn a new trade or hobby, set a habit of practicing 20 minutes each day.
- **Exercise**: Even short exercises—push-ups, crunches, or walks—can boost mood and health.

Start small. Trying to flip your life all at once can be overwhelming. Pick one or two habits you want to focus on. When they feel natural, add another.

---

7. Avoiding Old Patterns

Bad habits formed before or during prison might still pull at you. These can include sleeping until midday, hanging around aimlessly, or filling your time with activities that bring no real benefit. A stable routine helps block these tendencies. If you have a plan for your day, you are less likely to be drawn into harmful boredom.

Also, watch out for triggers that lead to old patterns—like certain areas or people that remind you of crime or substance use. If you know you waste time with negative influences, structure your day so you are busy during those times, or avoid those people if possible.

---

8. Keeping Health a Priority

Physical and mental health are crucial for a fresh start. Include some form of self-care in your daily or weekly routine:

- **Meal Planning**: Try to include fruits, vegetables, and proteins. You do not have to be a chef—simple, balanced meals are enough.
- **Exercise**: This can be as simple as a 20-minute walk, some push-ups, or light dumbbell work at home. Regular movement helps with stress and overall energy.
- **Sleep Schedule**: Aim for a set bedtime and wake-up time. In prison, lights-out might have been forced. Outside, it is your call. Lack of sleep can lead to mood swings and poor decisions.
- **Mental Breaks**: If you feel overwhelmed, take five minutes to breathe slowly or step outside for fresh air. Sometimes writing in a journal or talking to a supportive friend can ease your mind.

9. Staying on Top of Obligations

Depending on your legal status, you might have to attend probation appointments, drug tests, or therapy sessions. You may also have child support or other legal payments to make. Make these obligations part of your core routine:

1. **Mark the Dates**: Put the appointments in your calendar. Set reminders a day or two ahead.
2. **Plan Your Route**: If you need public transport, check schedules in advance to avoid being late.
3. **Communicate**: If there is a conflict (like a job interview at the same time), call your officer or the person in charge as soon as possible. Do not just skip the appointment.

Missing legal obligations can lead to bigger problems. By weaving them into your weekly routine, you stay on top of them and avoid unpleasant surprises.

10. Handling Changes in Routine

Life is unpredictable. Sometimes your schedule will be disrupted—maybe you get a new job shift, or a family emergency happens. A strong routine can handle changes if you remain flexible. Consider these steps:

- **Adjust Quickly**: If your shift changes from morning to evening, rewrite your daily plan. Move your personal tasks to earlier or later slots.
- **Stay Calm**: Large changes can be stressful. Do not fall into panic. Instead, think logically about how to rearrange your day.
- **Prioritize**: If you have to drop something due to time limits, let it be something less crucial. For example, skip a TV show rather than skipping your counseling session.

Having a routine does not mean being rigid. It means you know what is important and can adapt when reality shifts.

11. Evening Wind-Down

A good evening routine can help you rest better and wake up feeling fresh. Some ideas:

- **Set a Cut-Off for Electronics**: Phones, TVs, and games can keep you awake. Try to turn them off 30–60 minutes before bed.
- **Prep for Tomorrow**: Lay out clothes, pack a lunch, or organize your bag if you need one for work or appointments. This saves morning stress.
- **Reflect on Your Day**: Think about what went well and what was hard. This reflection can guide small improvements for the next day.
- **Bedtime Ritual**: Some people like a short shower, reading a light book, or listening to calm music. It signals your brain that it is time to sleep.

Getting enough sleep is vital for clear thinking and emotional balance. If you find yourself staying up too late, try setting an alarm to remind you it is bedtime.

---

12. Time Management Skills

You can sharpen your time management by:

1. **Estimating Task Duration**: If you know a chore takes 30 minutes, schedule that block of time. Do not pretend it only takes 10, or you will run late.
2. **Chunking Tasks**: Group similar tasks together. For example, do all your calls or emails in one block.
3. **Avoiding Procrastination**: If a task can be done now and it only takes a few minutes, do it. Delaying every little chore can lead to a huge load later.
4. **Leaving Buffers**: Allow extra time between tasks or appointments. If you plan everything back to back, one delay can ruin your whole schedule.

With better time management, you feel less rushed and can handle unexpected events more calmly.

---

13. Including Positive Social Activities

Routines should not be all work and no fun. You can schedule time to connect with friends or groups in healthy ways:

- **Weekly Meet-ups**: Maybe every Friday evening you see a friend for coffee or a meal.
- **Group Activities**: If you belong to a sports club, church, or support group, mark their events on your calendar. This ensures you keep up with social contacts.
- **Phone Check-Ins**: Set a routine to call a family member once a week if you cannot see them in person.

These regular social interactions can keep loneliness at bay and help you stay grounded. Just make sure they do not conflict with your work or other critical duties.

---

14. Tracking Your Progress

If you really want to see the power of routines, track your progress over time. You can:

- **Keep a Journal**: Write down daily or weekly notes on what you accomplished, what frustrated you, and what you would like to do better.
- **Use a Habit Tracker**: Some people make a simple chart with days of the week. They check off whether they did their chosen habit (exercise, reading, cleaning) each day.
- **Note Improvements**: When you see how often you keep up with your habits, you may notice improvements in mood, finances, or relationships.

Tracking progress can motivate you to stick with routines. It also shows where you might need to adjust. For instance, if you always skip your planned 8:00 p.m. exercise, maybe that slot is not good, and you need to try early morning.

---

15. Breaking Down Big Goals into Small Steps

If you have a large goal—like saving money, getting a certain certification, or losing weight—you can feel overwhelmed. Routines help you break it down. For example:

- **Goal**: Save $2,000 in a year.
  - **Daily/Weekly Step**: Put aside $5 each day or $35 each week. Cut one small spending habit (like daily soda) and put that money in a savings jar.
- **Goal**: Earn a trade certificate in welding.
  - **Daily/Weekly Step**: Practice welding basics for 30 minutes if you have equipment, or study written materials each evening. Attend one class a week if offered locally.

By focusing on small daily or weekly actions, the big goal does not seem impossible. Over time, small steps add up.

---

16. Being Mindful of Triggers and Stress

Life after prison can come with triggers that spark anger, anxiety, or sadness. A well-structured routine can cushion you from these emotions. For instance, if you know the evening hours make you restless, plan a calming activity (light exercise, a puzzle, or reading). If certain memories surface at night, keep a journal by your bed to jot down thoughts instead of letting them swirl in your head.

If stress gets high, do not toss your routine aside. Instead, adjust it. Maybe you need an extra break during the day. Or you might need to talk to someone in your support circle. The routine is there to support you, not to box you in.

---

17. Adapting Routines for Shift Work

Not all jobs are 9-to-5. If you work the night shift or have rotating shifts, creating a routine can be trickier. You might sleep during the day and be awake at odd hours. Still, plan your "morning" routine whenever you wake up, and your "evening" routine whenever you go to sleep. The concept stays the same: a set sequence of actions that prepare you for work and rest.

If shifts change often, you can create a flexible template. For example, your day always starts with a small meal, a shower, and a quick check of to-dos, no matter if that's at 6:00 a.m. or 6:00 p.m.

---

18. Avoiding Overcommitment

It is easy to pack your day with too many tasks, thinking you must do everything at once. But overcommitment leads to burnout. If you are juggling a job, counseling sessions, family duties, and personal goals, you have to be realistic. It might be better to do fewer tasks well than to do everything poorly.

Set boundaries. If friends constantly want your time during your rest periods, politely explain you need some downtime. If you have children, you might rotate responsibilities with a partner or relative, so you are not carrying it all alone.

---

19. Rewarding Yourself in Simple Ways

Maintaining a routine might feel repetitive. You can keep yourself motivated by small rewards. For example, after a solid week of following your plan, treat yourself to a favorite (but modest) snack or activity. It does not have to be expensive—maybe a favorite movie at home, or an afternoon walk in a park.

These small rewards give you something to look forward to. They mark the fact that you stuck to your plan. Over time, the benefits of the routine—like less stress, better health, and progress toward goals—become their own reward. But a little treat now and then does not hurt.

---

20. Conclusion of Chapter 8

Routines might not sound exciting, but they offer a powerful tool to reshape your life after prison. By choosing a consistent wake-up time, scheduling tasks, and balancing work with personal needs, you set yourself on a smoother path. The daily rhythms keep you busy with good habits and prevent old destructive patterns from creeping back.

Even on days when you do not feel motivated, a strong routine can carry you forward. You do not have to think hard about what to do next because you have a plan in place. Over time, you will see that regular habits—waking up early, exercising a bit, planning your meals, tracking your money—add up to major improvements in your lifestyle.

When life changes, adjust your routine rather than abandoning it. These patterns should serve you, not trap you. By staying organized, looking after your health, and including room for social connections, you build a life that is both stable and flexible. And stability is crucial when you are determined to stay out of trouble and make a new way for yourself.

Yes, it takes effort at first to set up these daily patterns. But once they become normal, you might wonder how you ever lived without them. Building a routine is like laying down railroad tracks for your day: you decide where they lead, and then you just follow the rails you have set. This kind of order can bring peace of mind and a sense of solid ground under your feet—two things that help you keep moving ahead.

Chapter 9: Looking After Your Physical Health

Physical health is a major piece of building a stable and positive life after prison. Feeling strong and well can help you stay focused on your goals, keep a better mood, and handle daily challenges without wearing yourself out. In prison, your health care might have been limited, and life on the outside gives you new choices and responsibilities. This chapter looks at how to form simple habits that keep your body healthy, where to find affordable medical help if needed, and how to guard against common health pitfalls that people face after release.

---

1. Why Good Health Matters After Prison

When you feel strong in your body, you also tend to feel stronger in your mind. You can concentrate more easily, stay calm under pressure, and have better energy for work or family time. Poor health, on the other hand, can open the door to low mood or stress. If you are fighting constant headaches, body aches, or diseases that go unchecked, it is harder to follow all the other advice—like getting a job, managing your anger, or meeting parole rules.

Also, good health can keep you from old habits. Some men get back into substance use to handle physical pain or general fatigue. By looking after your health, you lower the temptation to mask discomfort with harmful actions. It is easier to choose a better path when your body is not dragging you down.

---

2. Building a Basic Fitness Routine

You do not have to join an expensive gym to stay in shape. Think about how you moved your body in prison—maybe you did push-ups in your cell or walked laps in the yard. You can continue similar routines outside:

1. **Walking**: If you live near safe sidewalks or a park, walking can strengthen your heart, lungs, and legs. Start with 15 minutes a day and gradually increase.
2. **Bodyweight Exercises**: Push-ups, squats, sit-ups, and planks can build strength without special equipment. You can do them at home or in a local park.

3. **Light Jogging or Running**: If your knees and joints are okay, running can be a good way to burn off stress and calories. Go at a slow pace to avoid injury.
4. **Sports or Recreation**: If you enjoy basketball, soccer, or any other activity, see if there is a local group you can join. This also helps you meet people in a healthier setting.

Try to exercise at least three days a week. If that is too much at first, aim for two. Over time, you can add more. Small and consistent efforts beat doing extreme workouts that you cannot stick with.

---

3. Staying Flexible and Avoiding Injury

Some men focus on heavy workouts but forget to stretch or warm up. That can lead to strains and injuries. A few tips:

- **Warm Up**: Before any serious exercise, do five minutes of easy movement—like marching in place, shoulder rolls, or light arm circles.
- **Stretch**: After you exercise, do simple stretches for your legs, arms, and lower back. Hold each stretch for about 15 seconds, but do not bounce.
- **Listen to Your Body**: If you feel sharp pain, stop that exercise. There is a difference between normal muscle soreness and pain that signals injury.
- **Rest Days**: Your muscles need time to recover. Try not to do the exact same heavy workout every single day. You can switch muscle groups or do lighter activities like walking.

These steps protect you from injury, which can set you back for weeks if you push too hard too soon.

---

4. Eating Better on a Tight Budget

You do not need fancy or expensive foods to eat in a healthier way. There are budget-friendly steps to improve your meals:

1. **Buy Basics in Bulk**: Rice, beans, oats, and other staples are often cheaper when bought in larger bags. These can form the base of many meals.
2. **Frozen or Canned Vegetables**: They are often less expensive than fresh produce and still offer vitamins. Look for low-salt versions if you can.

3. **Simple Proteins**: Eggs, canned tuna, beans, or cheaper cuts of chicken can give you the protein you need. You do not need steak or fancy fish every day.
4. **Avoid Sugary Drinks**: Soda and energy drinks can drain your money and add extra sugar. Water is free (or very cheap if you need to buy it in some areas) and much better for your body.
5. **Cook at Home**: Eating out costs more. A big pot of soup with beans, vegetables, and some meat can last several meals. You can freeze leftovers to eat later.

If you have not done much cooking before, start simple. Practice a few recipes that use cheap, healthy items. Over time, you will learn to prepare meals that taste good and do not cost a lot.

---

5. Managing Weight and Overall Health

After prison, it is common for men to experience sudden changes in weight, either gaining or losing. Handling your weight is not just about looking a certain way—it is about avoiding health problems like heart disease or diabetes.

- **Track Portions**: Pay attention to how much you eat at each meal. It is easy to overeat when a lot of food is available, especially if you used to feel hungry in prison.
- **Drink Water**: Sometimes thirst can feel like hunger. Have a glass of water first if you think you want a snack.
- **Aim for Balance**: A balanced plate might have a protein (meat, eggs, beans), some veggies, and a carb source (rice, whole grain bread, or potatoes).
- **Limit Junk Food**: Chips, sweets, and fast food can be okay once in a while, but not every day. They can cause weight gain and leave you feeling tired.

If you have a medical condition like high blood pressure or diabetes, follow the dietary advice from your doctor. Even small changes—like switching from white bread to whole wheat—can make a difference.

---

6. Dealing with Substance Use Risks

If you used drugs or alcohol before prison, your body might be more at risk if you start using again. Some men also turn to new substances outside because of stress or peer pressure. Think carefully about the consequences. Substance misuse can destroy your health, your relationships, and your freedom.

- **Look for Healthier Coping Ways**: If you feel stressed, try exercise, talking to a trusted friend, or practicing calming techniques (deep breathing, short walks, or writing in a journal).
- **Seek Support**: If you feel a strong urge to use substances, connect with a counselor, a 12-step group, or a local recovery program.
- **Keep Clean Surroundings**: Avoid social groups that center around drug or heavy alcohol use. That environment can make it much harder to stay clean.

Physical health includes staying free from things that harm your body. Substances can also aggravate mental health issues, making it harder to stay on track with your goals.

---

7. Getting Regular Checkups

Even if you feel healthy, it is wise to see a doctor or clinic once a year for basic checkups. They can catch problems early, like high cholesterol or pre-diabetes, before they turn serious. If you have a history of certain conditions—such as high blood pressure, hepatitis, or certain infections—follow up with the recommended tests.

Where to Go for Low-Cost or Free Care

- **Community Health Centers**: Many towns have sliding-scale clinics that charge based on your income.
- **Health Departments**: County or city health offices may offer free screenings or immunizations.
- **Nonprofit Clinics**: Some charities or religious groups run free clinics.
- **Veterans Affairs (VA)**: If you served in the military, you might be eligible for VA health services.

If you are on parole or probation, ask your officer if they know about local programs. Sometimes they have lists of free or reduced-cost health resources.

8. Dealing with Stress-Related Aches and Pains

Men who have been in prison often carry stress in their bodies, resulting in headaches, back pain, or tight muscles. If your job is physically demanding—like construction or warehouse work—this strain can worsen. Consider these options:

- **Stretching and Massage**: You can do basic stretches at home. Sometimes gently rubbing your own shoulders, neck, or lower back can ease tight spots.
- **Hydration**: Dehydration can cause muscle cramps and headaches. Drink enough water, especially if you work in heat or do physical labor.
- **Physical Therapy**: If you have an old injury, a physical therapist can give you specialized exercises. This might cost money, but it can prevent bigger health costs later.
- **Rest and Sleep**: Chronic lack of sleep can increase body aches. Strive for 7–8 hours of rest each night if possible.

Persistent pain is a signal to pay attention. Do not ignore it or just take painkillers. Figure out the cause and see if changes in posture, exercise, or rest can help.

9. Staying Aware of Infections and Diseases

Life in prison can expose you to certain infectious diseases. Outside prison, you might face different hazards. It is wise to practice good hygiene to avoid spreading or catching illnesses:

- **Hand Washing**: Wash with soap for at least 20 seconds, especially before meals and after using the restroom.
- **Cover Coughs and Sneezes**: Use your elbow or a tissue.
- **Safe Intimacy**: Protect yourself and your partner by using precautions if you are sexually active.
- **Watch for Symptoms**: If you have a fever, persistent cough, rash, or unusual body changes, get medical advice. Early treatment can stop problems from getting worse.

10. Keeping a Simple Health Record

Track important health details in a small notebook or digital file. You might record:

- **Dates of Checkups**
- **Blood Pressure Readings**
- **List of Medications**
- **Notes on Any Chronic Conditions**
- **Allergies or Past Surgeries**

This helps you remember everything if you switch clinics or need emergency care. You can also note how you feel day-to-day—like if a certain food causes stomach trouble or if a certain exercise gives you joint pain. Having a written record can help doctors pinpoint issues faster.

---

11. Getting Dental and Eye Care

Teeth and vision are often ignored, but they can be big factors in your overall well-being:

- **Dental**: Untreated tooth decay can lead to infections, intense pain, and expensive procedures. Look for low-cost dental clinics. Brush twice a day and floss daily if you can.
- **Eye Exams**: If you have blurred vision, headaches from reading, or eye pain, an exam can reveal if you need glasses or have an eye condition. Some places offer free basic eye screenings.

Good dental health also helps with employment, as missing or painful teeth can affect how you speak or your confidence in public-facing jobs.

---

12. The Role of Rest and Relaxation

Health is not just about workouts and diet. You also need time to unwind. Chronic stress can raise blood pressure, disrupt sleep, and lead to mental strain. Healthy relaxation can include:

- **Quiet Time Alone**: Sitting calmly for a few minutes, listening to soothing music, or doing light stretches.
- **Relaxation Exercises**: Simple breathing exercises (inhale for four counts, exhale for four counts) can calm your mind.
- **Hobbies**: Activities like painting, writing, or tinkering with small projects can give your mind a break from worries.
- **Nature**: Spending time outside, whether it is a local park or a safe natural area, can reduce stress.

When you make rest a regular part of life, your body and mind can recover from daily demands more easily.

---

13. Preventing Return to Unhealthy Habits

If you used unhealthy coping methods in the past—such as binge eating, avoiding medical care, or doping yourself to handle pain—be alert for signs you are slipping. Maybe you notice yourself skipping meals all day then eating loads of junk at night. Or perhaps you feel tired but keep pushing yourself without rest. If that old pattern resurfaces, take these steps:

1. **Identify the Trigger**: Are you bored, stressed, or dealing with conflict?
2. **Replace the Habit**: Go for a short walk or call someone supportive if you feel the urge to fall into old behaviors.
3. **Seek Professional Help**: If you are overwhelmed by health concerns, see a doctor or counselor. It is better to get help early than wait until you are in crisis.
4. **Revisit Your Goals**: Remind yourself why you want to stay healthy—maybe for your family, for stable employment, or just to avoid feeling sick all the time.

---

14. Emotional Health Ties into Physical Health

Emotional well-being has a direct effect on how your body feels. Stress, depression, or anxiety can make you tired, give you headaches, or worsen chronic conditions. If you notice emotional struggles:

- **Consider Counseling**: A mental health professional can teach you coping tactics.

- **Use Your Support System**: Share your feelings with a friend, mentor, or group member.
- **Practice Good Self-Talk**: Avoid beating yourself up with negative words. Encourage yourself as you would a friend.
- **Stay Active**: Physical movement can release chemicals in your brain that boost your mood.

Even something as simple as talking out your worries can help you avoid physical stress symptoms.

---

15. Choosing Healthier Surroundings

Sometimes your living environment is beyond your control. But if you can, pick or shape your surroundings to support health:

- **Clean Home**: Keep your place free from clutter, trash, or pests. A tidy space helps you avoid health hazards like mold or bugs.
- **Smoke-Free Spaces**: If you do not smoke, try not to be in places with heavy secondhand smoke. If you do smoke, think about quitting or at least cutting down to reduce lung strain.
- **Safe Air and Water**: If your tap water is questionable, use a water filter or boil water before drinking. Good air flow (like opening a window) can also help if your area's air quality is decent.

Your body responds to the environment you live in. Even small improvements—like sweeping floors regularly—can keep you healthier.

---

16. Handling Work-Related Risks

Some jobs are rough on the body—construction, factory work, or jobs with heavy lifting. Protect yourself:

- **Use Proper Techniques**: Lift with your legs, not your back. Ask for help if an object is too heavy.
- **Wear Safety Gear**: If the job site requires gloves, goggles, or steel-toe boots, use them. Ignoring safety rules can lead to injury or job loss.
- **Take Short Breaks**: If allowed, do quick stretches every couple of hours. This keeps muscles from locking up.

- **Communicate**: If equipment is faulty or conditions are unsafe, tell a supervisor or union rep (if you have one). Do not risk your health by staying silent.

Your long-term physical health can be damaged by daily unsafe practices. Be proactive about staying safe on the job.

---

17. Finding Low-Cost Health Insurance (If Needed)

If you do not have health insurance through an employer, consider government programs or marketplace plans:

- **Medicaid**: If your income is very low, you might qualify.
- **Low-Cost Clinics**: Some clinics treat uninsured patients at reduced fees.
- **Health Insurance Marketplace**: Depending on where you live, you might get subsidies that lower your monthly insurance cost.

Medical bills can pile up fast without coverage. Even a basic plan can protect you from huge bills if you need emergency care.

---

18. Sticking to a Regular Sleep Schedule

One of the biggest health mistakes men make after prison is flipping their sleep schedule. Maybe they stay up late watching TV or hanging out, then feel groggy all day. Good sleep supports everything else:

- **Set a Bedtime**: Choose a time that lets you get 7–8 hours before your wake-up alarm.
- **Limit Caffeine Late in the Day**: Coffee or energy drinks after mid-afternoon can keep you up at night.
- **Create a Wind-Down Period**: Turn off bright screens, dim the lights, and do something relaxing for 30 minutes before bed.
- **Keep It Cool and Dark**: If possible, keep your sleeping space a bit cool and without bright light. Use curtains or blinds if streetlights shine in.

A steady sleep routine helps your body repair itself, supports weight control, and makes you more alert at work or in daily tasks.

19. Checking In with Yourself

Take a few minutes every day or week to ask: "How do I feel physically? Am I run-down, in pain, or lacking energy?" If you feel a drop in your usual strength or notice a new ache, do not ignore it. Look for reasons:

- **Not Enough Water**?
- **Not Eating Balanced Meals**?
- **Exercising Too Much or Not Enough**?
- **Feeling Unusually Stressed**?

This quick self-check can prevent small issues from growing into big health setbacks. If something feels seriously wrong, seek medical help.

20. Conclusion of Chapter 9

Taking care of your physical health might feel like another task on a long list, but it is actually a key part of staying free and building a better life. A healthy body can handle stress and daily challenges more easily, giving you a stable base to meet your goals—like holding a job, supporting your family, or simply feeling better day by day.

No matter how tight your budget, there are ways to eat more wisely, do basic workouts, and find low-cost medical help. Good health habits can protect you from harmful spirals, such as turning to substances or neglecting your well-being until you end up in the hospital. Simple steps, done regularly, can lead to big benefits over time.

Remember, it is never too late to focus on your health. Even if you did not care about it before or during prison, you can start now. Each walk, healthier meal, and doctor visit is an investment in your future. A well-cared-for body can support a determined mind, and together they can help you keep moving forward.

Chapter 10: Strengthening Relationships with Family and Friends

One of the hardest parts about leaving prison can be rebuilding connections with loved ones. You might have lost touch while you were locked up or missed important moments—birthdays, graduations, or even family hardships. On top of that, people's feelings about your past actions can be complicated. But a strong support network of family and friends can give you emotional strength, practical help, and a sense that you belong somewhere.

This chapter talks about practical ways to renew your ties with family members, rebuild friendships, and create healthier relationships. You will learn how to handle guilt, set boundaries, and communicate so that you do not push away the people who matter most.

---

1. Why Relationships Matter

Having people who care about you can keep you grounded when life gets tough. A family member might let you sleep on their couch for a night, or a friend might connect you to a job lead. Emotional support also gives you a reason to stay out of trouble. If you know loved ones rely on you, you may be less tempted to return to the lifestyle that led you to prison.

Relationships are not just about what you can get, though. Giving back to the people who stuck by you shows gratitude. This exchange builds stronger bonds and makes everyone feel valued.

---

2. Dealing with Regret or Shame

You might feel ashamed of the harm you caused before going to prison. This shame can make you avoid certain relatives or friends. While it is good to admit your mistakes, disappearing from people's lives will not fix anything. A better approach might be:

- **Acknowledge Past Wrongs**: A short and direct apology can be the first step. "I know I messed up and I am sorry."

- **Show Positive Change**: Words mean less if you still act the same way. Follow through with consistent behavior—like keeping a job, staying sober, and being trustworthy.
- **Give People Space**: Some folks may still be angry or uncertain. Let them process their feelings at their own pace, and do not force them to forgive you overnight.

Shame is a strong feeling, but letting it keep you isolated only makes things worse. Transparency and honest effort can start the healing process.

---

3. Reaching Out After a Long Gap

If you have not talked to certain family members or friends for a while, start small. You might send a simple text: "Hi, I have been thinking of you and hope you are well. I am working on improving my life. If you are open to talking, I would love to catch up." Keep it short and respectful. Some will respond positively, some might not respond at all, and some might be hostile.

If you get a negative reaction, do not argue or get defensive. Just let them know you understand their feelings. Anger from them could be a sign that they were deeply hurt. Over time, consistent growth on your part might change their view.

---

4. Communication Basics

Good communication can fix or prevent many problems in relationships:

1. **Listen Actively**: When a loved one speaks, do not just wait for your turn. Show you are hearing them by nodding, repeating important points, or asking clarifying questions.
2. **Use Calm Words**: If things get tense, avoid shouting or name-calling. Instead, say how you feel: "It hurts me when…" or "I feel stressed because…"
3. **Stay on Topic**: If you are discussing finances, do not bring up old fights about something unrelated. Keep the conversation focused on the issue at hand.
4. **Apologize When Needed**: If you say something hurtful, correct yourself quickly. A simple "I am sorry, that was out of line" can cool down a heated moment.

This approach may take practice, especially if you learned to communicate differently in prison. But open, respectful communication is the backbone of healthy relationships.

5. Setting Boundaries with Family

Sometimes family members can be overbearing or may engage in behaviors that pull you in the wrong direction. Setting boundaries protects you and them. A boundary can be:

- **Time**: You only visit certain relatives for a short period if extended time leads to arguments.
- **Location**: You do not go to a relative's home if you know there is drug use there.
- **Topics**: You refuse to engage in topics that always lead to shouting matches. If they bring it up, you calmly change the subject or excuse yourself.

Boundaries are not about cutting people off. They are about keeping the relationship in a healthy zone so you can remain on track. Communicate your boundaries clearly. If someone refuses to respect them, you might have to reduce contact for your own well-being.

6. Rebuilding Trust with Loved Ones

Trust is not automatic after prison. Your actions might have hurt or worried others. You can rebuild trust with steady reliability:

- **Keep Your Promises**: If you say you will call at 6:00 p.m., call at that time. If you promise to pay back a small loan next week, do it.
- **Be Honest**: Do not hide stuff out of fear. If you slip up or have a tough time, be upfront rather than lying. People can handle the truth better than betrayal.
- **Show Respect**: Even small things—like cleaning up after yourself or offering help around the house—show you value the relationship.
- **Consistency**: Trust grows when your new behavior lasts for weeks, months, or years. Do not expect immediate acceptance. Give them time to see you have changed.

7. Parenting and Reconnecting with Children

If you have kids, time in prison might have strained the bond. Depending on their age, they might feel confused or resentful. Steps to reconnect:

1. **Take It Slowly**: Children might not welcome you with open arms right away, especially if they are used to you being absent.
2. **Apologize Simply**: Kids may not understand deep explanations. A simple "I am sorry I was gone. I care about you very much" can mean a lot.
3. **Show Up**: If you say you will attend a school event or weekend meetup, be there. Consistency matters even more for children than for adults.
4. **Respect the Other Parent or Caregiver**: If your child lives with someone else, cooperate with them. Avoid arguments in front of the child.
5. **Spend Quality Time**: Even small moments—like coloring together, kicking a ball, or reading a short story—help rebuild bonds.

If you are dealing with legal custody issues, follow court orders. Keep your cool, and show the court that you are stable and capable of being a good parent.

8. Dealing with Friends Who Are Still in Crime

Some friends from before might still be involved in illegal activities. Hanging around them can land you back behind bars. It is okay to care about them, but you must protect your own freedom:

- **Be Clear About Your Limits**: Explain that you will not participate in crime or be around it. If they respect you, they will not push you.
- **Suggest Better Outlets**: Invite them to do something lawful, like playing sports or joining a community event. If they scoff, that is a sign you might need to part ways.
- **Do Not Let Guilt Trap You**: You might feel bad for leaving them behind, but remember your future depends on staying away from trouble.
- **Stay Polite**: You do not have to be hostile or rude. A calm, respectful approach is often best. But be firm.

Think carefully about each friend. Some might be ready to change. Others might drag you down. Choose wisely, because your friends' actions can affect your own path.

9. Creating New Friendships

Making new friends after prison can be daunting, but it is possible:

- **Join Community Events**: Check out local meetups, sports leagues, or free classes. You might share an interest with someone and start a friendship.
- **Volunteer**: Helping at a food pantry or charity event can bring you into contact with people who value service and positive action.
- **Workplace Bonds**: Over time, you may become friendly with coworkers who have good habits. Just take it slow—learn who they are before sharing personal details.
- **Online Groups**: Be cautious, but you can find groups focused on your interests, like cooking, hiking, or cars. Look for people who live nearby, then meet in public places if you decide to connect in person.

New friendships can provide fresh perspectives and reduce the pull of old negative social circles. Aim for people who motivate you to keep growing.

10. Handling Relatives Who Create Conflict

Sometimes a family member has a negative pattern—they might shame you constantly, bring up old fights, or spread rumors. You can try these steps:

1. **Calm Discussion**: Tell them how their behavior affects you. They might not realize how hurtful they are.
2. **Propose Solutions**: Suggest talking about certain topics only with a neutral person present. Or ask them to bring up concerns in a calmer way.
3. **Use Boundaries**: If they refuse to change, limit your contact. That might mean shorter visits or only seeing them at larger family gatherings so you are not one-on-one.
4. **Seek Mediation**: If you live in the same household, a family counselor could help. Some community centers offer low-cost sessions.

You cannot force a relative to act kindly, but you can protect your own well-being by deciding how and when you interact with them.

11. Balancing Old Ties and New Life

Building a new, stable life does not mean you must abandon everyone from your past. But you do need to decide which ties are healthy and which ones are harmful. People who knew you when you were involved in crime might have trouble accepting your new choices. Some might mock you for staying legal. Others might admire your transformation.

- **Respect Yourself**: You have a right to change. Do not let anyone guilt you into regressing.
- **Give People a Chance**: If an old friend is curious about living better, share your insights. Maybe you can motivate them too.
- **Protect Your Progress**: If someone tries to drag you into illegal schemes, remember the stakes. Your freedom and future matter more than fitting in with old friends.

---

12. Consistency and Patience in Relationships

People you care about might have been disappointed many times. They might test you to see if you really have changed. That can be frustrating, but it is normal. Remain consistent:

- **Keep Showing Up**: If you agreed to meet someone at a certain time, do it.
- **Avoid Anger**: If they bring up your old mistakes, do not explode. Stay calm and remind them you are focusing on better actions.
- **Be Reliable**: If you say you will call, call. If you say you will help with a chore, get it done.

Over months or even years, this steady behavior speaks louder than any speech about how you have changed.

---

13. Practicing Forgiveness

You might need to forgive family members who did not support you when you were locked up. Or you might hold bitterness towards a friend who never wrote you or visited. Holding grudges can poison your mind. Forgiveness does not mean you let them walk all over you. It means you stop holding onto the anger that harms you.

- **Reflect**: Ask yourself if clinging to resentment helps you or hurts you.
- **Decide**: Choose to let go of the grudge, even if you do not fully forget.
- **Set Healthy Boundaries**: You can forgive someone but still keep a bit of distance if needed for your own peace.

Forgiving can free your mental energy for better things. It is a step toward peace within yourself.

---

14. Celebrating Good Moments Together

Healthy relationships thrive on positive shared moments. You do not need fancy parties. Even a simple meal can bring warmth if you enjoy it together. When something good happens—like landing a new job or finishing a training program—invite your loved ones to share a small treat, watch a movie, or just talk about the success. These moments help bond you and remind everyone that life is moving in a better direction.

---

15. Using Technology to Stay Connected

If you live far from your family, technology can help:

- **Video Chats**: Services like Zoom, Google Meet, or FaceTime let you see each other's faces.
- **Group Messages**: You can have a group chat with siblings or close friends to share updates quickly.
- **Social Media**: Carefully use it to keep in touch, but watch out for negative or triggering posts. Mute or unfriend people who cause unnecessary drama.

Technology is not a full replacement for in-person visits, but it keeps bonds alive when meeting face to face is tough.

---

16. Coping with Loss

You might learn that someone you cared about passed away while you were in prison, or that a relationship ended. Dealing with grief can be intense. Talk to trusted friends or a counselor about the pain. Do not feel like you have to handle it alone. Letting out sadness or regret can be part of healing. Also, give yourself time to mourn. For some men, planting a tree or writing a letter to the lost loved one (even if they will never read it) can provide a form of closure.

---

17. Family Gatherings After Prison

Events like holidays or reunions can be stressful. People might ask tough questions or make remarks. Some tips:

1. **Prepare Mentally**: Decide how you will answer if someone asks about prison or your record. Keep it brief and factual if you do not want to share too much.
2. **Pick Allies**: Have a relative or friend there who knows your situation and can steer conversations away from uncomfortable topics if needed.
3. **Set Limits**: If the atmosphere becomes hostile, it is okay to leave.
4. **Look for Good Moments**: Try to find a few family members you can talk to peacefully. Focus on those connections rather than the negative ones.

---

18. Strengthening Ties Through Mutual Help

Sometimes the best way to rebuild a relationship is by helping each other. For instance:

- **Offer Assistance**: If your sister needs help moving furniture or your uncle needs a ride to an appointment, lend a hand if you can. Actions often speak louder than words.
- **Ask for Their Knowledge**: Maybe a relative is good with budgeting, car repairs, or cooking. Let them teach you. This shared time can ease tensions and create new positive memories.
- **Start Small Projects**: Team up with a friend or family member to fix up a backyard, paint a room, or volunteer somewhere. Working side by side can bond you without the pressure of heavy talk.

People often connect more deeply when they cooperate on tasks rather than just sitting around trying to find something to say.

19. Knowing When to Walk Away

Not every relationship can be mended. If someone is abusive, constantly trying to involve you in crime, or deeply disrespectful of your new life path, you may need to let that relationship go, at least for now. This decision can be painful, especially if it is a close family member. But staying in a toxic situation can drag you back into trouble or destroy your self-esteem.

- **Be Honest**: Say something like, "I want a better life, and our interactions are hurting that. I need space."
- **Focus on What You Can Control**: You cannot make them change, but you can remove yourself from their harmful influence.
- **Keep the Door Open** (If You Wish): Let them know you are willing to reconnect if they decide to respect your boundaries and stop unhealthy behavior.

---

20. Conclusion of Chapter 10

Strengthening your bonds with family and friends is a vital step in creating a life that keeps you away from prison and toward genuine progress. This process may involve apologizing, setting firm boundaries, and learning to communicate in better ways. You may face rejection or anger from some people at first, but consistent positive behavior can shift their minds over time.

Remember, relationships are a two-way street. You cannot force someone to forgive or welcome you back. But you can consistently show that you are no longer the person who hurt them. You can ask for forgiveness in a clear and humble way. You can also offer your own forgiveness for those who let you down.

At the end of the day, people are social beings. We need connection and acceptance. When family and friends see you handling stress in healthier ways, holding a steady job, and keeping your word, their trust might rebuild. This new trust can give you a sense of belonging and motivation. Whether it is your children, siblings, parents, or old buddies, nurturing positive ties can be an anchor that keeps you from drifting back to the life you left behind.

It will not always be smooth or simple. Some relationships may remain broken or distant, and that is reality. But each healed connection can enrich your life and give you a sense of hope. Step by step, you can build a circle of people who genuinely support you, helping you walk the path of true growth rather than slipping into the traps that once held you down.

Chapter 11: Managing Stress in Everyday Life

Stress is a normal part of life. Everyone experiences it, whether they have been to prison or not. But for men who have spent time behind bars, stress can feel more intense because they might be juggling more responsibilities—finding a job, following parole conditions, rebuilding family relationships, and handling day-to-day worries. If stress is not handled well, it can lead to anger, health problems, or even bad decisions that put a person at risk of going back to old ways.

In this chapter, we look at practical steps for recognizing stress, dealing with it in a healthy manner, and creating a calmer environment for yourself. We also address how to spot when stress is becoming harmful and what to do about it before it grows out of control.

---

1. What Is Stress?

Stress is your body's reaction to pressure or demands. It can come from outside sources, like a demanding boss or a noisy environment. It can also come from the inside—your own worries, fears, or expectations. A certain amount of stress can be helpful, pushing you to meet deadlines or solve problems. But too much stress, or stress that never goes away, harms both your mind and body.

Common signs of stress include:

- Feeling tense or jumpy
- Trouble sleeping
- Mood swings or irritability
- Headaches or stomach aches
- Feeling overwhelmed, like there is too much on your plate

When these signs appear, it is a signal that you need to step back and handle things differently.

---

2. Recognizing Your Stress Triggers

A "trigger" is something that sets off your stress response. For one person, it might be loud noises or big crowds. For another, it might be money worries, arguments with a partner, or deadlines at work. Write down the situations that make you feel pressured or nervous. This can help you see patterns.

Some common stress triggers after prison include:

1. **Legal Obligations**: Meetings with parole officers, fear of messing up a condition.
2. **Financial Struggles**: Not having enough money to cover rent or bills, worrying about where to find a job.
3. **Relationship Tensions**: Arguments with family or friends, feeling misunderstood by loved ones.
4. **Social Stigma**: Knowing people might judge you if they learn about your record.
5. **Unpredictable Routines**: Struggling with disorganized schedules or sudden changes.

Once you know your main triggers, you can plan ways to reduce their impact or face them with better coping methods.

---

3. Healthy Ways to Lower Stress

There is no magic trick for stress relief. Instead, think of it like having a toolbox of small methods. When stress hits, you grab one or more of these methods to bring yourself back to a calmer state. Here are some ideas:

1. **Breathing Exercises**
    - Inhale slowly for four counts, hold for a second, then exhale for four counts.
    - Repeat a few times. Focus on the rhythm of your breath, not on the stressful thought.
2. **Physical Activity**
    - A short walk can help clear your head.
    - If you like more intense activities, do push-ups, squats, or a quick run.
    - Physical movement releases body tension and can shift your mood.
3. **Writing It Down**
    - Take five minutes to write out what is bothering you.

- Sometimes just naming the problem on paper makes it feel more manageable.
- You can also write down possible solutions and pick one to try.

4. **Short Breaks**
    - Step away from the stressful situation if possible.
    - Even a brief moment in a quiet spot can help you think more clearly.
5. **Stay Hydrated and Nourished**
    - Dehydration and hunger can raise stress levels.
    - Drink water and eat balanced meals. Low blood sugar can worsen anxiety and irritability.
6. **Music or Calming Sounds**
    - Listening to soothing music or nature sounds can help slow your heart rate.
    - Keep a set of headphones handy if you have them, so you can tune out a chaotic environment.

Over time, you will find which methods work best for you. Some men lean on breathing exercises, others prefer physical outlets. The key is to practice these methods regularly, not just when stress becomes overwhelming.

---

4. Organizing Your Day to Cut Down Stress

A big source of stress is feeling like life is chaotic and you cannot keep up. This is where routines (as discussed in Chapter 8) can help. By planning your day, you avoid a lot of sudden crises. Here are some tips:

- **Create a Weekly Schedule**: Write or type out your obligations (work shifts, parole meetings, bills due). Knowing what is coming lets you prepare.
- **Use Alarms and Reminders**: If you have important appointments, set alerts on your phone or mark them on a calendar.
- **Avoid Last-Minute Rushes**: If you must be somewhere at 9:00 a.m., plan to leave earlier than you think you need to. This prevents the stress of traffic or unexpected delays.
- **Time Blocks**: Group similar tasks together. For instance, handle all calls or emails in one block of time rather than scattering them throughout the day.

When your schedule is organized, you free your mind from constantly worrying about what you might be forgetting. That alone can lower stress significantly.

5. Setting Realistic Goals

It is good to have targets for yourself—like saving a certain amount of money, finding a better job, or training in a new skill. But if you set goals that are too big and try to reach them too quickly, you can burn out. Stress piles up when you feel you are always behind. Here is a better approach:

1. **Break Goals into Steps**: If you want to save $1,000, think about how much you can realistically put aside each week, maybe $20. In about a year, you will get there.
2. **Celebrate Small Wins (In a Simple Way)**: When you hit a milestone, note it as progress. For example, "I saved $100. That is a tenth of my big goal."
3. **Adjust as Needed**: If life throws you a curve, do not panic. Just adjust the plan. Maybe it will take a bit longer than you hoped, but steady progress is still progress.

By focusing on reachable steps, you reduce the stress of feeling you have an impossible mountain to climb.

6. Talking to Someone You Trust

Keeping stress bottled up can make it worse. If you have a friend, family member, or mentor who is open to hearing about your worries, lean on them. Even a quick conversation can clear your head. They might have ideas you have not considered. Or maybe they just provide a listening ear, which can ease the pressure.

- **Choose Carefully**: Open up to someone who respects your privacy and will not spread your personal details around.
- **Be Direct**: Say something like, "I am feeling really tense about money right now, and I need to talk it through."
- **Return the Favor**: When they need someone to listen, be there for them too.

If you do not have someone you trust, consider a counselor or a support group. Many places have low-cost or free options for people who need to talk. Getting professional advice is not a sign of weakness; it is a practical step to safeguard your well-being.

---

7. Using Humor and Simple Enjoyment

Laughter actually helps lower stress hormones in the body. If you can find a reason to smile or chuckle, it can calm you down. You might watch a funny clip online, read a comic, or recall a fun memory. The idea is not to ignore your problems but to give your mind and body a short break from tension.

Similarly, small pleasures—like having a cup of tea, working on a hobby, or playing with a pet—can reset your mood. These positive activities act like small stress buffers throughout the day.

---

8. Avoiding Unhealthy Coping Methods

Sometimes men turn to harmful ways to deal with stress—like alcohol, drugs, or gambling. These might give short-term relief, but they create bigger problems in the long run:

- Substance use can lead to addiction, money issues, and even a violation of parole.
- Gambling can drain your finances and cause more stress.
- Avoiding problems (like ignoring bills) just piles them up until they explode.

If you notice yourself leaning toward these habits, recognize that it is time to seek help. Reach out to a counselor, a recovery group, or a trusted friend who can guide you to a better path. Remember, you left prison to build a healthier life, not trade one cage for another.

---

9. Knowing When Stress Turns into Something More

Normal stress can be managed with the steps above. But sometimes stress morphs into serious conditions like severe anxiety or depression. Watch out for signs that might suggest professional help is needed:

- Feeling hopeless most days
- Losing interest in activities you used to enjoy
- Trouble sleeping for more than a couple of weeks
- Thoughts of harming yourself or not wanting to live
- Constant worry that keeps you from functioning

These signs do not mean you are weak. They mean you might need more specialized support—like therapy, medication, or a mental health program. Talk to a doctor or counselor if you suspect your stress has gone beyond normal levels.

---

10. Stress in the Workplace

Holding down a job can be stressful, especially if you are new to it or dealing with demanding tasks. Some tips:

- **Organize Your Tasks**: Make a quick list each morning of what needs to be done. Mark the tasks that are most urgent.
- **Communicate**: If your boss or coworkers are piling too much on you, talk to them politely. Maybe you can ask for clearer instructions or more realistic deadlines.
- **Take Short Breaks**: A quick stretch or a minute of deep breathing can keep stress from building up.
- **Separate Work and Home**: If possible, avoid bringing work stress home. When you clock out, try shifting your focus to personal or family life.

Handling job stress well can improve your performance and help you keep that steady paycheck.

---

11. Balancing Multiple Responsibilities

Many men leaving prison must juggle jobs, parole visits, family duties, classes, or counseling. That is a lot to handle at once. To avoid meltdown:

1. **Prioritize**: Figure out which things must be done first. For example, you cannot miss a parole appointment because it could lead to big trouble.
2. **Use a Calendar**: Write or type all your responsibilities and their due dates. Check this daily to see what is next.

3. **Say No When You Must**: If someone asks you to take on something extra and you are already swamped, it is okay to say no. Overloading yourself leads to stress and mistakes.

By staying aware of your limits, you respect your own need for downtime and reduce stress-related errors.

---

12. Mindset Shifts

Sometimes stress comes from how we view problems. If you believe every setback is the end of the world, you create more tension. Adopting a realistic mindset can reduce stress. This includes:

- **Seeing Problems as Challenges**: Instead of "This is impossible," think, "This is tough, but I can find a way through."
- **Accepting What You Cannot Change**: Some things—like certain parole rules—are out of your control. Accepting them rather than fighting them in your mind can lower stress.
- **Recognizing Progress**: You are not the same person you were in prison. Each day you stay on the right path is proof you are moving forward.

A balanced mindset does not pretend everything is perfect. It just acknowledges that you can handle more than you might think, especially if you take it step by step.

---

13. Physical Health Ties to Stress

Poor physical health can make stress feel worse (see Chapter 9). If you are always tired or in pain, small problems can push you over the edge. Keep an eye on:

- **Sleep Quality**: Chronic lack of rest makes it harder to cope with daily challenges.
- **Nutrition**: A steady supply of nutrients helps regulate mood and energy levels.
- **Exercise**: Moving your body can burn off stress chemicals.
- **Addictions**: Smoking, heavy drinking, or drug use might give brief relief but add long-term stress to your body and life.

When your body is better cared for, your mind can handle pressure more effectively.

---

14. Creating a Calming Environment

Your surroundings can either calm you or add to your tension. If possible:

- **Keep Your Living Space Tidy**: A messy home can make you feel overwhelmed.
- **Add Soothing Touches**: If you can, place some simple decorations or items that bring a feeling of peace—a nice poster, a plant, or a comfortable chair.
- **Manage Noise**: Loud and constant noise can spike stress. Use earplugs or low-volume background music if needed.
- **Set Boundaries with Others**: If you have roommates or family members who stress you out 24/7, create times and spaces where you can have quiet.

A calm environment does not have to be fancy or expensive. Even a small, clean corner can give you a sense of retreat.

---

15. Relying on Support Networks

Earlier chapters stressed the value of friends, family, and community groups. These networks are also a shield against stress. If you are nearing your breaking point, a good support network can offer a shoulder to lean on or practical help:

- A friend might lend you a bit of money to cover a bill so you do not panic about it.
- A mentor can remind you of coping strategies when you feel lost.
- A group session can show you that you are not alone in struggling with stress after prison.

It is easier to handle pressure when you know others have your back.

---

16. Handling Sudden Crises

Life sometimes throws unexpected hurdles—like a sudden job loss, an eviction notice, or a family emergency. These moments can skyrocket your stress. Here is a way to approach them:

1. **Stay Calm**: Take a few deep breaths before you react.
2. **Assess the Situation**: What exactly is the problem? Write it down if it helps.
3. **List Possible Actions**: Brainstorm solutions or steps you can take.
4. **Reach Out**: Call someone in your support network or a professional who can guide you.
5. **Take Action Step by Step**: Tackle what you can control. Even small moves can reduce the feeling of chaos.

It is easy to panic, but panic rarely solves anything. Slowing down just enough to plan your response can prevent an emergency from turning into a total meltdown.

---

17. Giving Yourself Permission to Rest

Some men push themselves nonstop out of fear that they are "behind" everyone else because of time spent in prison. While hard work is good, never resting can lead to burnout. Give yourself permission to pause:

- **Schedule Breaks**: If you work eight hours, allow yourself a short break every couple of hours to clear your head.
- **Plan a Day Off**: If possible, have one day a week for lighter tasks or relaxation.
- **Engage in Low-Key Activities**: Even reading a book for fun or taking a slow walk can refresh you.

Rest is not laziness; it is part of taking care of your overall well-being.

---

18. Building Confidence in Your Coping Skills

The more you handle stress successfully, the more confident you will become. Each time you choose a healthy way to respond instead of getting angry or giving up, you prove to yourself that you have changed. Keep track of these small victories:

- Maybe you faced a tough conflict at work but talked it out calmly.
- Perhaps you had a big bill due but managed it by calling a friend for help or speaking with the billing office for a payment plan.
- Maybe you felt overwhelmed but used deep breathing and avoided a meltdown.

Write these successes down in a small journal. On tough days, look back at them and see how far you have come.

---

19. Long-Term Stress Management Plans

It is not enough to handle stress once in a while. You need an ongoing plan to keep it in check:

1. **Make Stress Checks Part of Your Routine**: Each morning or evening, ask, "Am I feeling stressed? Why?"
2. **Update Your Tool Kit**: If certain methods (like walking or writing) stop working as well, try new ones (like stretching, guided audio exercises, or arts and crafts).
3. **Stay Honest**: If your stress levels are getting worse despite your efforts, talk to someone or seek professional support before it gets out of hand.

By seeing stress management as an ongoing part of life, you can avoid letting small tensions snowball into big breakdowns.

---

20. Conclusion of Chapter 11

Stress is a normal, unavoidable part of living, especially for men who are rebuilding their lives after prison. But it does not have to control you. By noticing the signs of stress early, knowing your triggers, and using healthy coping strategies, you can keep stress at a manageable level. An organized schedule, realistic goals, and a supportive network go a long way in preventing stress from ruling your day.

If you ever find yourself drowning in pressure, remember the simple steps: breathe, step away if you can, talk it out, and tackle problems one at a time. Build positive habits—like regular exercise, balanced eating, and enough rest—and stay watchful for signs that stress is turning into something more serious. With practice, you will learn to navigate life's ups and downs without being overwhelmed. This control over stress can help you keep your freedom, hold your job, and continue the progress you have made since leaving prison.

Chapter 12: Dealing with Moments That Remind You of Prison

After spending time behind bars, certain sights, sounds, or situations in the outside world can bring up unwanted memories. These moments—often called "triggers" or "flashbacks"—can spark anxiety, anger, or even shame. They might appear suddenly, like hearing a door slam that sounds like a prison gate, or noticing a guard-like uniform that reminds you of correctional officers. Coping with these triggers in a safe way is important for your emotional health and your progress outside.

This chapter explains how to handle these troubling reminders of prison life. We look at why they happen, how to deal with them in the moment, and ways to gradually reduce their power over you.

---

1. Understanding Triggers Related to Prison

Prison can be a tense environment where you are constantly on edge. Even after leaving, your mind may still react to stimuli linked to life behind bars. These triggers might include:

- The sound of keys jingling (like guards' keys)
- Doors slamming
- Loud arguments or fights nearby
- Being in a cramped space that feels like a cell
- Seeing uniforms that resemble prison guards or officers
- The smell of certain cleaning chemicals used in prison

Triggers happen because your brain connected these cues with intense fear, stress, or survival instincts in prison. Now, when you encounter something similar, your body and mind might react as if you are still there.

---

2. Recognizing the Signs of a Prison Flashback

A flashback is more than a simple memory. It can involve physical sensations or intense emotional responses. You might:

- Feel your heart pound
- Start sweating or breathing quickly
- Feel sudden anger or panic
- Want to escape the area immediately
- Mentally see or hear parts of prison life, as if you are reliving them

Not everyone experiences full flashbacks. Some just feel uneasy or restless without immediately realizing what caused it. Learning to link these feelings to the trigger helps you cope faster.

---

3. Grounding Techniques to Bring You Back to the Present

When a trigger hits and you feel trapped in the memory of prison, grounding methods can help you return to the present moment. These techniques anchor you in what is real around you:

1. **Name Five Objects**
   - Look around and quickly name five objects you see.
   - This forces your mind to focus on what is actually in front of you right now.
2. **Senses Check**
   - Notice one thing you can see, one thing you can smell, one thing you can hear, and one thing you can touch.
   - Shifting your attention to real-world input calms the flashback.
3. **Breathe and Count**
   - Take a slow breath, then count to four. Exhale, count to four.
   - Repeat several times, focusing on the counting rather than the memory.

These steps help remind your brain that you are not in prison anymore, even if your body is reacting like you are.

---

4. Facing Triggers Gradually

Some triggers cannot be avoided forever. For example, if your job requires you to go through secure doors that slam shut, you may hear a similar sound as in prison. Rather than live in constant anxiety, you can learn to face the trigger in small steps:

1. **Plan a Strategy**
   - If you know a door will slam, remind yourself it is just a door and you are free to leave the building anytime.
   - Practice a grounding technique beforehand.
2. **Desensitization Over Time**
   - Repeated exposure to the trigger, while you stay calm, can reduce its power.
   - Each time you hear the door but keep your cool, you are teaching your mind that this sound is no longer a threat.
3. **Seek Support**
   - If certain environments are too intense at first, ask a trusted friend to accompany you.
   - Having someone else there can remind you that you are safe now.

---

5. Talking About Prison Memories in a Safe Space

Bottling up these memories can make them grow stronger. Finding a counselor, support group, or even just one trusted friend who understands can help:

- **Share Bits at a Time**: You do not have to spill every painful memory in one go. Talk about one aspect of prison life that affects you now.
- **Ask for Understanding**: Explain to your friend or counselor how certain sounds or sights make you feel. This way, they will know why you might react strongly.
- **Listen to Others**: If you are in a group with people who also have prison memories, their experiences might give you ideas on how to cope.

Talking about it does not erase the past, but it can soften its grip on your everyday life.

---

6. Using Relaxation Methods When Triggers Strike

An intense trigger or flashback can feel overwhelming. Relaxation methods can settle your body's stress response:

- **Progressive Muscle Relaxation:**
  - Tense a muscle group (like your fists or shoulders) for a few seconds, then slowly release.

- - Move to another muscle group. This reduces overall tension.
- **Visualizing a Safe Place**:
  - Close your eyes and picture a calm spot—like a quiet beach or a peaceful park.
  - Imagine the sounds, smells, and sights there until you feel your body calm down.
- **Stretching**:
  - Roll your shoulders, stretch your arms overhead, or bend and gently reach for your toes.
  - This simple act can release tightness brought on by stress or fear.

Pick one or two methods that appeal to you and practice them regularly, even when you are not triggered, so they come naturally when you need them most.

---

7. Mindset Shifts About Past Experiences

Some men feel stuck in shame or anger about their prison time. That can intensify triggers. While you cannot change the past, you can change how you view it:

- **Acknowledge It**: "Yes, I was in prison, and it was a tough environment."
- **See Your Growth**: "I am no longer there, and I have learned lessons that I can use to live better."
- **Accept What You Cannot Erase**: Punishing yourself mentally each time a trigger hits only adds more pain. It is okay to feel upset about your history, but also give yourself credit for trying to move on.

By shifting your inner narrative from "I am ruined by prison" to "I survived prison and now I am shaping my future," you reduce the emotional weight of memories.

---

8. Practical Steps to Avoid Over-Stimulation

Sometimes triggers become worse in places that overload your senses—like very crowded areas, loud concerts, or chaotic events. If you find these situations too intense:

1. **Plan Your Exits**
   - Know where you can leave if it gets overwhelming.

- Stand near the edge of a crowd, not in the center.
2. **Use Headphones**
    - If loud noise triggers you, consider using noise-canceling or regular headphones in busy environments.
    - Play calming music or even white noise to block out stressful sounds.
3. **Limit Your Time**
    - If you must be in a busy place, decide on a short time frame.
    - Give yourself breaks—step outside for fresh air if needed.

These little steps give you more control. Feeling trapped or powerless can bring back prison memories. Ensuring you have an "escape route" can ease that tension.

---

9. Handling Unexpected Triggers

Not all triggers are predictable. You might hear a random sound that makes you jump, or see a stranger who looks like a guard. In these moments:

- **Stop for a Second**: If you can, pause and take a deep breath.
- **Identify the Trigger**: Realize, "Oh, this is reminding me of prison."
- **Ground Yourself**: Use a quick technique—count something around you or focus on your breathing.
- **Shift Your Thought**: Tell yourself, "I am free now. This is not a threat."

Being caught off guard can feel embarrassing or frustrating, but remember that these responses are normal after a high-stress experience like prison. With practice, you can recover faster each time.

---

10. Building New Positive Associations

One way to weaken old triggers is to build new, positive associations with similar sights or sounds. For example, if the sound of keys rattling bothers you, you can:

- Hold your own keys and jingle them while doing something pleasant, like watching a comedy show or chatting with a friend.
- Over time, your mind might stop linking that sound only to guards and tension, and start linking it to normal daily life or even positive moments.

This is a form of retraining your brain. It can take time, but it can be very effective.

11. When to Seek Professional Help

If prison memories and triggers are causing severe anxiety, nightmares, or flashbacks that disrupt your life, it might be time to see a mental health professional. Some signs include:

- Constant nightmares or trouble sleeping
- Avoiding important places or activities because of fear of triggers
- Feeling numb or disconnected from reality for long stretches
- Experiencing panic attacks that you cannot control

A therapist experienced with post-traumatic stress or similar conditions can teach specialized methods—like trauma-focused therapy or EMDR (Eye Movement Desensitization and Reprocessing)—to help you process prison memories in a safer way.

12. Talking with Others in Similar Situations

Sometimes, friends or family members have not been behind bars and cannot fully grasp the triggers you face. Joining a group of people who also spent time in prison can create a sense of understanding:

- They might share what triggers them and how they cope.
- Group support can reassure you that you are not alone or "crazy" for experiencing these memories.
- You can compare notes on local resources, like counselors who specialize in reentry trauma.

Check local community centers or nonprofit reentry programs to see if there are support groups specifically for men who have been to prison.

13. Controlling Anger Related to Triggers

Some triggers cause anger instead of fear. Maybe hearing a guard-like voice makes you want to lash out because you remember feeling degraded. In these moments, controlling that anger is crucial:

1. **Pause and Name It**: "I am feeling angry because this reminds me of how guards treated me."
2. **Breathe Before Responding**: Give yourself time to calm your heart rate.
3. **Channel the Energy**: If anger does not subside, try a quick physical outlet—ten push-ups or stepping outside for a brisk walk.
4. **Self-Talk**: Remind yourself that the current situation is different from prison. You do not need to defend yourself in the same way you did then.

By handling anger constructively, you avoid harming your progress outside prison.

---

14. Balancing Acceptance and Change

It is important to accept that some memories will remain. You cannot erase all reminders of prison. At the same time, you can change how strongly you react to them. This balance looks like:

- **Accepting Reality**: "Yes, I was in prison, and these triggers exist."
- **Working on Coping**: "But I can learn to calm myself and reduce their power."

Resisting or denying your past can keep you stuck. Embracing the fact that it happened (but not letting it define your whole life) allows you to move forward.

---

15. Handling Dreams or Nightmares About Prison

For some men, the triggers come at night in the form of dreams. You might wake up sweating, your heart racing, convinced you are still locked up. If this happens often:

- **Create a Pre-Bed Routine**: Spend 10 minutes doing something calming, like reading a light book or listening to gentle music.

- **Limit Heavy Topics Before Sleep**: Try not to watch intense prison shows or argue about stressful issues right before bed.
- **Jot Down Dreams**: Keep a simple notebook. Write down the nightmare briefly. Sometimes putting it on paper helps your mind let it go.
- **Use a Grounding Technique**: If you wake up in panic, do the senses check or breathe deeply to remind yourself you are in a safe bed, not a prison cell.

If nightmares do not improve, a mental health professional might help you with specific tools to reduce them.

---

16. The Role of Forgiveness in Letting Go

Part of dealing with prison triggers can involve feelings of hatred or bitterness—maybe toward guards, the system, or even yourself. Holding onto this bitterness can keep triggers alive. Consider steps to forgive where you can:

- **Identify the Source**: Who or what are you angry at? A guard who mistreated you? The judge who gave you a longer sentence? Yourself for making bad choices?
- **Decide if Forgiveness Is an Option**: Forgiveness does not excuse what happened, but it frees you from dwelling on it.
- **Release the Grudge**: You may not talk to those people again, but you can stop letting their actions poison your thoughts every day.

Forgiveness is a personal choice. It does not make you weak. It can be a way to break the chain that ties you to the past.

---

17. Building Positive New Memories

One of the best ways to move beyond prison triggers is to fill your life with fresh, positive experiences. Each happy or successful moment can overshadow some of the painful ones:

- **Try New Activities**: Pick up a skill, join a community sports league, or explore a hobby that intrigues you.

- **Invest in Relationships**: Spend time with supportive friends or family doing enjoyable things—like cooking together, playing board games, or visiting local parks.
- **Set Achievement Milestones**: Whether it is completing a training program or keeping a job for six months, note these steps as proof that your life is bigger than your prison past.

Over time, your brain will attach more meaning to these new memories, making the prison recollections less dominant in your daily life.

---

18. Respecting Your Own Pace

Healing from the mental and emotional impact of prison is not a one-week fix. It can take months or years. You might feel fine for a while, then get hit by a strong trigger unexpectedly. That does not mean you are back to square one. It means the process continues:

- **Be Patient**: Give yourself credit for every small improvement.
- **Track Your Progress**: Maybe you used to freak out every time you heard a door slam, but now it only bothers you occasionally. That is progress.
- **Seek Help If You Slide Back**: A brief setback is not failure. Connect with a counselor or a friend if you feel stuck again.

Recovery is like building a muscle. You get stronger with consistent effort, even if some days feel harder than others.

---

19. Creating a Personal Emergency Plan

If you fear a trigger might push you to do something destructive (like lash out violently or run away from a stable situation), prepare a plan:

1. **List Warning Signs**: Note how you feel or act when you are about to lose control (sweating, shaking, yelling).
2. **Steps to Take**: For example, "Step outside and call my mentor," or "Go to the bathroom and run cold water on my face, then do deep breathing."
3. **Emergency Contacts**: Write down phone numbers of one or two people you can call if you are in crisis.

4. **Safe Places**: Identify a location you can go where you feel calmer—a friend's house or a quiet park.

Having this plan written down and easily available can prevent panic or harmful reactions in a tough moment.

---

20. Conclusion of Chapter 12

Moments that remind you of prison can feel like a chain pulling you back to a place you want to leave behind. But triggers and flashbacks do not have to rule your life. With grounding exercises, the right mindset, and possibly professional guidance, you can learn to face these reminders without letting them disrupt your progress.

Accept that certain sounds, sights, or smells might always bring a twinge of memory. Yet, each time you practice a coping method, you show yourself that you are not helpless. You are now in control, living in a world where you have choices and freedom. Over time, the power those triggers hold can lessen. By building a life full of positive experiences, caring relationships, and honest work toward self-improvement, you replace the dark echoes of prison with a new outlook.

This does not happen overnight, and setbacks may occur, but each step you take in confronting triggers weakens their control over you. In moving forward, you continue the work of shaping a healthier, safer life for yourself—far away from the walls that once held you.

Chapter 13: Handling Money and Building a Budget

Money problems can cause huge stress, especially for men who have left prison and are trying to rebuild their lives. When you are short on cash, it is easy to fall back into bad habits or illegal ways of getting money. But with the right knowledge and tools, you can take control of your finances, even if your income is small at first. In this chapter, we look at how to create a simple budget, avoid common traps, and build a more stable financial future step by step.

---

1. Why Money Management Matters After Prison

When you are locked up, many daily expenses are covered or managed for you: food, a place to sleep, and certain medical needs. Outside, you have to pay for all these things yourself. On top of that, you might have parole fees, child support, or other legal financial obligations. Good money management helps you handle these costs without feeling completely overwhelmed.

It also protects you from the panic of not knowing if you can pay your rent or put food on the table. A clear budget plan can reduce stress and keep you away from risky shortcuts. Employers, landlords, and even banks often look at how stable you are with money. Showing that you can manage a paycheck responsibly helps open more doors, like getting a decent place to live or eventually qualifying for a car loan.

---

2. Understanding Income and Expenses

A budget is basically a way of tracking two things:

1. **Income**: How much money is coming in. This could be from a job, side gigs, government benefits, or any other source.
2. **Expenses**: How much money is going out. This covers rent, food, transportation, bills, personal items, and so on.

When you spend more than you make, you go into debt or end up with no money by the end of the month. That can lead to late fees, eviction, or even desperation that might push you back into illegal activities. The goal is to keep your spending equal to or less than your income so that you stay in control.

---

3. Setting Up a Simple Budget

You do not need complicated spreadsheets to begin. A piece of paper or a basic notebook will do:

1. **List Your Income**
    - Write down all the money you expect to get in one month. Include paychecks, part-time side jobs, or any aid you receive.
2. **List Your Fixed Expenses**
    - These are costs that stay the same each month, like rent, car payment, or a phone bill. Write each one next to how much it costs.
3. **List Your Variable Expenses**
    - These costs may change from month to month—like groceries, gas, or electricity. Write down an estimate for each.
4. **Calculate the Difference**
    - Subtract total expenses from total income. Hopefully, you get a positive number or zero. If you get a negative number, that means you are spending more than you have.

At first, just do your best guess. Over a few months, you will see where your money actually goes, and you can adjust. The key is honesty. Do not write "groceries: $50" if you really spend $150. That will only cheat yourself.

---

4. Tracking Actual Spending

It is one thing to write a budget. It is another to stick to it. For at least a month or two, try to track every dollar you spend. This might feel tedious, but it can open your eyes to where your money really goes:

- **Keep Receipts**: Stuff them in an envelope or snap photos with your phone.
- **Write Down or Type Entries**: Each night, note what you spent and on what. Even if it was just $2 for a soda.

- **Compare to Your Budget**: At the end of the week, see if you are matching your planned amounts or going over in certain categories.

This process can be a "golden gem" because it reveals spending leaks. You might notice you are spending $30 a week on snacks that you did not plan for. That is $120 a month—enough to pay part of a utility bill or save for a better phone. Knowing this helps you tighten up your budget.

---

5. Cutting Back on Unnecessary Costs

When you see your spending in black and white, you may find areas you can reduce. Here are some tips:

1. **Look at Food Spending**
    - Eating out regularly can drain money fast. Cooking at home usually costs less.
    - Plan meals in advance so you do not buy food on impulse.
2. **Check Your Subscriptions**
    - Do you pay for streaming services, music apps, or a gym you do not use? Consider canceling or finding cheaper options.
3. **Avoid Expensive Habits**
    - Cigarettes, alcohol, or gambling can eat up a big chunk of cash. Cutting back or quitting can save a lot.
4. **Shop Smart**
    - Buy store-brand items instead of name brands.
    - Check clearance racks or used goods if you need clothes or household items.

Even small changes add up over time. If you manage to save $20 here and $10 there each week, by the end of the month, you might have enough to handle a bill or put a bit into savings.

---

6. Dealing with Debt and Past Fines

Many men come out of prison with debts—like court fines, restitution, or unpaid child support. Ignoring these does not make them go away. In fact, interest and penalties can pile up. Try the following:

- **Contact the Office in Charge**: If you owe court fines, call the court clerk. If you owe child support, call the agency. Ask about a payment plan or reduced amounts based on your current income.
- **Be Honest About Your Income**: Do not promise huge monthly payments you cannot afford. If you default on a payment plan, it can cause more trouble.
- **Check for Programs**: Some nonprofits help with legal fees or can negotiate with courts to lower your fines if you show you are making an effort.

Taking action shows you are responsible. It may also protect you from random wage garnishments (where they pull money from your paycheck) or even an arrest if you ignore court orders.

---

7. Avoiding Quick Money Traps

When money is tight, you might see ads or hear suggestions for "fast" solutions, like payday loans, car title loans, or get-rich-quick schemes. These can be very dangerous because of high interest rates and hidden fees:

- **Payday Loans**: You borrow a small amount against your next paycheck but end up paying huge fees, which can trap you in a cycle of debt.
- **Title Loans**: You use your car as collateral. If you cannot pay back on time, you lose your car.
- **"Guaranteed" Online Jobs**: Many are scams that charge you up front or steal your information.
- **Illegal Activities**: Returning to crime for fast cash is a direct route back to prison.

If a deal sounds too good to be true, it usually is. Talk to someone knowledgeable before you take a leap. Sometimes, waiting a bit or looking for an honest part-time gig is a safer path.

---

8. Building an Emergency Fund

An emergency fund is a small stash of money set aside for surprises—like car repairs, medical bills, or a sudden job loss. Even $300 to $500 can save you from panic and bad choices. Here is how to start:

1. **Set a Tiny Goal**: Aim for $100, then $200, and so on.
2. **Regular Small Contributions**: If you can, set aside $5, $10, or $20 each paycheck into a separate savings spot.
3. **Treat It as Off-Limits**: Do not use this money for daily expenses unless it is truly an emergency.

This fund grows slowly but gives you peace of mind. Without it, one unexpected crisis can push you back into financial chaos.

---

9. Banking Basics

Some men avoid banks because they fear hidden fees or worry about past mistakes. But having a bank or credit union account can protect your money from theft and help you build a financial record. Start with:

- **Checking Account**: This is for daily use—depositing paychecks and paying bills. Ask about low-fee or no-fee accounts. Some banks have "second chance" accounts for people with a flawed history.
- **Savings Account**: Good for your emergency fund or other goals. Savings accounts are not for constant withdrawals, so you earn a little interest and avoid dipping into it.
- **Direct Deposit**: Many jobs pay by direct deposit. This is safer than carrying a check around, and you get your money faster.

Be mindful of overdraft fees. If you spend more than you have, the bank might charge you a high fee. Keep track of your balance and set alerts if the bank allows it.

---

10. Creating Room for Personal Wants

A budget should cover needs first—rent, groceries, utilities, and any legal payments. But it is also important to have a little room for wants, like a small entertainment budget or a treat for yourself sometimes. If you do not allow any enjoyment, you might get frustrated and abandon your budget.

- **Set a Modest Amount**: Maybe $10 or $20 a week for something fun (like a streaming service or a meal out).

- **Stay Within That Limit**: If your "wants" money is gone, do not dip into rent or food money. Just wait until next time.

This helps you stick to your plan without feeling deprived. Over time, as your income grows, you can increase this fun category if you want.

---

11. Handling Financial Obligations to Family

Some men come out of prison owing relatives or friends who helped them with money. Others might have child support to catch up on. Handle these obligations with clarity:

- **Child Support**: Make an official payment plan or arrangement through the court. Even small, consistent payments show you are making an effort. If your income is very low, you might apply for a modification.
- **Personal Debts to Family or Friends**: Write out a simple agreement on how you will pay them back. For example, "I will give you $25 on the first of every month." Sticking to that plan shows responsibility and prevents conflict.
- **Avoid Secret Loans**: If a family member pressures you to borrow more or do something illegal to repay them, that is a red flag. Better to be honest that you cannot afford it than to put your freedom at risk.

---

12. Building Credit Wisely

Credit is a record of how reliably you pay back money. A good credit score can help you rent an apartment or get a car loan at a lower interest rate. But you must build credit carefully:

1. **Check Your Credit Report**
    - In some places, you can get a free credit report once a year. Look for errors or old debts that should be cleared.
2. **Pay Bills on Time**
    - Even small things like your phone bill matter if reported to credit bureaus. Consistency is key.
3. **Secure Credit Card or Store Card**

- If your credit is poor, you might start with a secured credit card (you deposit money as a security). Use it for small purchases and pay it off fully each month.
- Or get a low-limit store credit card if you can handle it responsibly.

Be careful not to overspend. A credit card is not free money. It is a loan you must repay on time to avoid interest and a damaged score.

---

13. Growing Your Income

Sometimes the best way to balance your budget is to earn more. You can:

- **Look for Overtime**: If your job allows it, extra hours can boost your paycheck. But avoid burnout.
- **Seek Better Jobs**: As you gain experience or training, apply for positions with higher pay. Keep building your skills.
- **Try Side Work**: Offer services like lawn care, painting, car washing, or small repairs in your neighborhood. If you do it well, word might spread and you can earn steady extra money.
- **Sell Unneeded Items**: Sometimes you have things you can sell online or at a yard sale.

Increasing income takes effort, but it can speed up debt repayment and savings. Just make sure you do it in a legal and sustainable way so you do not risk your freedom.

---

14. Keeping Financial Records

You do not have to be a perfect bookkeeper, but basic records help you stay on top of things:

- **Keep Key Documents**: Store pay stubs, receipts for major purchases, and any loan or rental agreements in a safe place.
- **Note Bill Due Dates**: Write them on a calendar or set phone reminders so you do not miss deadlines and get late fees.
- **Review Monthly**: Sit down once a month and check your budget against actual spending. Make adjustments where needed.

Clear records can also help if there is a dispute with a landlord or a billing error. You can show proof of what you paid or what was agreed.

---

15. Planning for Big Expenses

Over time, you might want or need larger purchases—a better car, a training course, or moving to a nicer place. Instead of jumping in without a plan:

1. **Research the Cost**: Find out how much it truly costs, including taxes, fees, or maintenance.
2. **Save Up**: Put aside money each week or month until you have enough for a solid down payment or full purchase.
3. **Compare Options**: If you are buying a used car, shop around and read reviews. Avoid shady dealers who prey on people with bad credit.
4. **Check Financing Terms**: If you borrow money, understand the interest rate and monthly payments. A bad financing deal can cost you big in the long run.

Thinking ahead can keep you from impulse buys or signing up for contracts you cannot handle.

---

16. Tips for Grocery Shopping on a Tight Budget

Food is a major expense, and it is easy to overspend if you do not plan. Consider:

- **Make a List**: Plan meals for the week and buy only what is on the list. This prevents impulse buys.
- **Shop Sales and Discounts**: If an item you regularly use is on sale, get a bit extra if you can store it.
- **Use Local Markets**: Sometimes produce is cheaper at local markets or discount grocery stores.
- **Cook in Batches**: Make a large pot of soup, chili, or stew and freeze portions. This saves time and money throughout the week.
- **Avoid Waste**: Use leftovers creatively. Tossing unused food is like throwing money away.

These strategies can significantly cut your monthly food bill and help you eat decently without going broke.

17. Dealing with Bill Collectors

If you are behind on payments, you might get calls or letters from collectors. This is stressful, but do not just ignore them:

- **Verify the Debt**: Ask for details in writing—amount owed, original creditor, etc. Some collectors try to make you pay for debts you might not recognize or no longer owe.
- **Negotiate**: You might offer a smaller lump sum or a manageable payment plan. Many collectors prefer getting something rather than nothing.
- **Stay Calm**: Collectors can be pushy. Know your rights. They cannot threaten to send you to prison over private debts (unless it is court-ordered fines or child support).
- **Get Help If Needed**: Some nonprofits offer free credit counseling. They can guide you in negotiating or consolidating debts.

Remember, ignoring the problem can lead to legal action or wage garnishment, so it is better to face it and try to work it out.

18. Building a Mindset of Responsibility

Managing money is not just about math. It is also about mindset. If you treat money casually or blame others for your hardships, you might not grow. Here are some attitudes to consider:

- **Own Your Financial Choices**: You decide where your money goes each day, even if your income is small.
- **Stay Patient**: Real change takes time. It may be many months before you see a big difference in savings or debt reduction.
- **Learn Constantly**: Keep picking up tips from friends, articles, or community classes.
- **Avoid Keeping Up with Others**: You might see someone flashing cash or buying fancy things. They might be deep in debt or involved in crime. Focus on your own plan.

This sense of personal responsibility keeps you grounded and motivated, even when it feels like progress is slow.

19. Planning for the Future

Once you have handled immediate issues, think long-term. Would you like to own a small business someday? Buy a house or condo? Retire without struggling? These are major goals. Start small:

- **Keep Growing Your Skills**: The more you can earn, the easier it is to reach bigger money targets.
- **Look Into Retirement Savings**: If your job offers a plan like a 401(k), consider putting a little in each paycheck. Time can help that money grow. If you are older, do what you can to build a small nest egg.
- **Teach Yourself More**: Learn about compound interest, investing in safe ways (like index funds or bonds), or other financial vehicles.

You do not need to be a finance expert. Small, steady steps can lead to a more comfortable life later on.

20. Conclusion of Chapter 13

Money can be a source of great stress or a tool for stability—it depends on how you handle it. After prison, you might start with a very tight budget, debts, and a low-paying job. But even with these challenges, you can create a plan that makes the most of every dollar. Tracking spending, cutting back on waste, and avoiding bad loans can save you from financial traps.

Over time, as you follow your budget, pay down debts, and maybe grow your income, you will notice more breathing room in your finances. That breathing room gives you freedom to make better decisions and handle emergencies without panic. You do not need to be rich to feel secure; you just need control over what comes in and goes out.

Yes, it takes patience to see real results. But each month of sticking to your plan builds better habits. Eventually, you might save for an emergency fund, pay off debts, or even start making moves to improve your future—like investing in education or learning a trade. Stay consistent, keep learning, and remember that every step away from financial chaos is a step toward a more stable and confident life.

Chapter 14: Setting Clear Goals for the Future

After prison, it is easy to get stuck just dealing with day-to-day problems—finding a job, paying bills, or meeting parole conditions. While these things are important, you also need a bigger direction for your life. Having clear goals gives you something to aim for, whether it is related to work, relationships, or personal growth. Without goals, you might drift or fall back into old habits. With goals, you have a roadmap that keeps you moving in a positive direction.

This chapter explores how to choose realistic goals, break them into doable steps, and stay motivated even when life throws challenges at you.

---

1. Why Goals Matter

Goals act like a lighthouse, guiding you toward a place you want to be. They can:

- **Give You Purpose**: Waking up each day with a clear aim helps you push through tough moments.
- **Focus Your Efforts**: Instead of wasting time or money, you channel your resources into actions that move you closer to your target.
- **Provide Hope**: Even if things are hard now, knowing you are working toward something better can keep your spirits up.
- **Measure Growth**: Goals let you see progress. You can look back and say, "I have come this far," which builds confidence.

People without goals often go through life just reacting to whatever happens. After prison, you likely want to shape a better path rather than just hope things turn out okay.

---

2. Picking the Right Goals

It is tempting to set massive targets, like "I want to be a millionaire in a year" or "I want to fix every mistake I ever made." But unrealistic goals can lead to frustration and quitting. Instead, focus on realistic yet uplifting aims. Think about:

- **Career/Work Goals**: Maybe you want to learn a trade, land a stable job, or start a small business someday.
- **Education Goals**: Getting a GED, finishing vocational school, or taking community college classes in a specific field.
- **Financial Goals**: Building savings, paying off debts, or improving your credit score.
- **Personal Growth Goals**: Learning better social skills, managing anger more effectively, or strengthening your self-image.
- **Family Goals**: Reconnecting with children, being a supportive partner, or helping a relative in need.

Pick a few areas that really matter to you. The best goals are ones that align with your values and your new life. They should be something you care about, not just what you think others expect.

---

3. The Power of Writing Goals Down

A "golden gem" many overlook is the act of writing or typing goals clearly:

- **Creates Clarity**: Turning a fuzzy idea into written words forces you to be specific.
- **Acts as a Reminder**: You can look at the written list each day or week to keep yourself on track.
- **Helps with Accountability**: If you share the list with a friend or counselor, they can check on your progress.

Try putting your main goals on a small piece of paper. Stick it where you will see it daily—like the inside of your closet door or a note on your phone's home screen. This constant reminder pushes you to stay active.

---

4. Breaking Goals into Manageable Steps

Big goals can feel daunting if you look at them all at once. That is why you break them down into smaller tasks:

1. **Define the Main Goal**: For example, "Get a commercial driver's license (CDL)."

2. **Identify Sub-Goals**: You might need to get a regular driver's license first if you do not have one, then study for the written CDL test, then save money for the training course, and finally pass the road test.
3. **Create a Timeline**: Assign rough dates for each step, even if they are just estimates.
4. **Track Completion**: Each time you finish a step, note it somewhere so you see progress.

With bite-sized steps, you are less likely to feel overwhelmed. Each small success also motivates you to tackle the next stage.

---

5. Using the S.M.A.R.T. Framework (If It Helps)

Some people use the S.M.A.R.T. method for goal setting:

- **S**pecific: Clearly define what you want (for instance, "Save $500 in three months," not "Save some money").
- **M**easurable: Set a number or clear marker so you can see if you are on track.
- **A**chievable: Make sure the goal is possible given your current situation.
- **R**elevant: Pick goals that match your bigger life vision.
- **T**ime-Based: Give yourself a deadline or target date.

You do not have to use this method, but it is a helpful template to make sure your goals are well-structured rather than just vague wishes.

---

6. Staying Motivated When It Gets Tough

Motivation does not remain high all the time. Sometimes you will feel tired, discouraged, or doubt yourself. Here are some ways to push through:

- **Remember Your "Why"**: Why did you choose this goal? Maybe you want a better life for your child or to prove to yourself you can succeed honestly. Keeping that reason in mind can spark renewed energy.
- **Visualize Success**: Spend a few minutes imagining how it will feel once you reach your target. This mental picture can energize you.

- **Reward Small Wins**: Each time you hit a milestone, do something simple to mark that step (like having a special homemade meal or spending an afternoon on a hobby).
- **Track Progress**: Keep notes or pictures showing how far you have come. That reminds you that every small action is adding up.
- **Seek Support**: When motivation dips, talk to a friend, mentor, or group who believes in your goals.

No one is motivated 24/7. The difference is that motivated people keep acting on their plan even on days they do not feel like it.

---

7. Balancing Multiple Goals

You might have more than one goal at once—like saving money, going to counseling sessions, and improving your relationship with family. That is fine, but be careful not to overload yourself. Focus on a small number of priorities so you do not get spread too thin.

- **Rank Your Goals**: Which ones are urgent and which ones can wait a bit? For example, finding stable work might come before planning a long-term business.
- **Plan Realistic Schedules**: Do not try to squeeze in five big tasks every single day. Make sure you allow time for rest, errands, and the unexpected.
- **Review Often**: Every month or so, see if you need to adjust. Maybe one goal is completed or no longer relevant, and you can shift focus to another.

Life after prison can be busy. Good planning prevents burnout and helps you move ahead in a balanced way.

---

8. Dealing with Fear of Failure

Some men fear setting goals because they worry about failing. They think, "If I do not try, I cannot fail." But that leads nowhere. A better approach is to see setbacks as part of learning:

- **Failing Forward**: If something does not work, ask yourself what went wrong and what you can do differently next time. This is how you grow.
- **Reducing High Stakes**: If a goal feels huge, make a practice run. For example, if you want to start a small car-washing service, you could first wash cars for free for relatives to perfect your process. Then, once you feel confident, charge paying customers.
- **Remember Past Successes**: Maybe you overcame addiction, learned a new skill, or survived tough prison conditions. You have already shown resilience.

Failure is not the end unless you stop trying altogether. Each attempt, even if imperfect, builds wisdom for the next try.

---

9. Adapting Goals as Life Changes

Life is unpredictable. You might set a goal to get a certain job, then find that job is no longer available. Or you might discover a new interest that excites you more. It is okay to adjust your goals:

- **Stay Flexible**: If circumstances change, sit down and update your plan. Maybe you aim for a similar position in a different company, or you pivot to a new idea.
- **Keep Core Values**: The details might shift, but the core of what matters—like honesty, growth, and stability—should remain.
- **Avoid Constant Changing**: Do not jump around too much or you will never complete anything. Give each plan a fair try before switching.

Being rigid can lead to frustration, while being too loose can lead to never finishing anything. Aim for a balanced approach that allows some changes without losing direction.

---

10. Enlisting Help and Mentors

You do not have to chase goals alone. Mentors or experienced folks in your community might guide you. For example:

- **Career Mentors**: Someone with experience in the trade or industry you want to enter. They can advise on training and job openings.

- **Community Support**: A local reentry program might have counselors who help set personal and professional goals.
- **Friends and Family**: Trusted ones can cheer you on or keep you accountable. Just make sure they are truly supportive.
- **Online Resources**: Many free tutorials, forums, and videos can teach you the basics of almost any skill—from car mechanics to coding.

Asking for help is not weakness; it is a smart move. Mentors often enjoy seeing someone willing to put in effort, and they may open doors you did not know were there.

---

11. Setting Goals for Personal Growth

Goals are not just about money or career. Personal growth can be just as important:

- **Health and Fitness**: Maybe you want to lose weight, gain muscle, or improve stamina.
- **Emotional Strength**: Learning better anger control (review Chapter 4), handling stress (Chapter 11), or working through regrets (Chapter 2).
- **Social Skills**: Becoming a better listener or learning how to resolve conflicts calmly.
- **Hobbies or Talents**: Playing a musical instrument, writing, drawing, or anything that enriches your life.

These goals might not bring direct cash, but they build self-worth and keep you away from negative influences. They can also fill your time with productive activities, reducing boredom that leads to bad choices.

---

12. Creating a Vision Board (If You Like Visuals)

Some people find a "vision board" helpful. It is a simple collage of pictures or words representing what you want in life. You can cut out images from magazines or print them, then glue them on a board or arrange them in a notebook:

- **Examples**: A photo of a house you want to rent or buy, a symbol of a trade certificate you aim to earn, or pictures of a happier family.

- **Place It Where You Can See It**: Each time you glance at the board, you remind yourself of the bigger picture.
- **Keep It Realistic**: While it is okay to have big dreams, focus on images that genuinely inspire you without being purely fantasy.

This method might seem silly to some, but for visual learners, it keeps motivation strong.

---

13. Handling Setbacks and Obstacles

No matter how well you plan, obstacles appear. You might lose a job, face a health issue, or have family problems that take time and energy:

- **Pause and Rethink**: Give yourself time to address the issue. You might need to slow down your progress on a certain goal while you resolve the crisis.
- **Do Not Abandon Your Main Aim**: Unless it becomes truly impossible, keep that end goal in mind. You might just adjust the timeline.
- **Seek Extra Support**: Hard times are when mentors, friends, or counselors can offer more help.
- **Practice Self-Compassion**: Blaming yourself harshly for every delay can sap your spirit. Acknowledge that life happens, and you can still get back on track.

Remember, a setback is not a sign that your goal was wrong. It is just part of the reality of life. The key is to adapt and keep going when you can.

---

14. Reviewing Progress Regularly

It is not enough to set goals and forget them. Check in with yourself:

1. **Weekly or Monthly Check-Ins**
   - Ask: "Am I doing the tasks I planned? Are they working?"
   - If yes, keep going. If no, figure out why.
2. **Celebrate (or Mark) Small Wins**
   - Notice what you have accomplished. For example, "I saved $100 more than last month."
   - Positive reinforcement helps keep you motivated.

3. **Adjust the Plan**
   - If you see a faster or better approach, switch. If you are behind schedule, maybe you need more time or a different strategy.

This constant review keeps your goals alive. It prevents the problem of setting big goals in January and forgetting them by March.

---

15. Keeping a Goal Journal

A goal journal can be a powerful tool. It is like a personal record of your journey toward improvement:

- **Daily or Weekly Entries**: Write down what steps you took, any progress or challenges.
- **Reflect on Feelings**: Note how you feel about the process—excited, frustrated, tired, etc.
- **Plan Next Actions**: End with what you intend to do tomorrow or next week.

Over time, reading past entries can show you how far you have come, remind you of lessons learned, and help you see patterns in your own behavior.

---

16. Handling Negative Influences

Even if you have clear goals, certain people or environments might drag you down:

- **Toxic Friends**: They might mock your goals or tempt you to skip steps.
- **Unsupportive Family Members**: They might bring up your prison past at every turn, making you doubt yourself.
- **Distracting Environments**: Places where you always end up wasting time or facing triggers (discussed in Chapter 12).

If possible, limit contact with those who constantly undermine your goals. Focus on spending more time in places or with people who respect your effort. This is not always easy, but your goals deserve a safe space to grow.

---

17. Balancing Confidence and Humility

While you should believe you can achieve your goals, watch out for arrogance. Sometimes people get a bit of success and start ignoring advice or breaking rules again. A healthy approach is:

- **Confidence**: "I can accomplish this if I keep working and learning."
- **Humility**: "I do not know everything. I can still learn from others or from my mistakes."

This balance keeps you open-minded and adaptable. It also helps you avoid repeating past errors that might land you back in trouble.

---

18. Celebrating (Marking) Milestones in a Meaningful Way

When you reach a milestone—like finishing a job training program or saving your first $500—take a moment to recognize it. You do not need a big party or fancy event. Simple ideas:

- Share the news with a supportive friend or mentor.
- Treat yourself to a small, budget-friendly item you have wanted.
- Write about how you feel in your goal journal.

This step matters because it shows you that progress is real. It also gives you energy to tackle the next phase. Just be careful not to blow your entire budget in the process.

---

19. Picturing Life Beyond the Basics

Once you have a steady job, some savings, and a calmer state of mind, you might wonder what is next. Goals do not have to end once you meet your initial targets. You can keep growing. Perhaps you want to:

- **Travel to a Nearby Place**: Even a small trip can expand your mind.
- **Learn Advanced Skills**: Maybe you can become a supervisor at work or start your own contracting business.
- **Contribute to Community**: Volunteer or mentor younger people at risk. Helping others can be a powerful way to reinforce your own progress.

Your life is not limited to "just getting by." You have the right to dream bigger if you wish, as long as you keep it realistic and remain consistent with your day-to-day responsibilities.

---

20. Conclusion of Chapter 14

Setting clear goals is a strong way to guide your life after prison. They give structure, purpose, and a way to measure how far you have come. Whether you want a better job, a healthier body, stronger family bonds, or simply more self-respect, defining those aims keeps you on track.

The process starts with picking goals that fit your real situation, then breaking them into smaller tasks. Write them down, track progress, and adapt as needed when obstacles appear. Lean on mentors, friends, or community support when your motivation dips. Avoid letting fear of failure or negative influences drive you off-course.

In the end, goals are not about perfection; they are about direction. Each small step you take toward them moves you away from the patterns that led to prison and toward a future you can be proud of. You do not need to rush or compare yourself to others. Just keep moving forward, one task at a time. Over the months and years ahead, these goals can reshape your life in ways you never thought possible when you were behind bars. Stay focused, stay patient, and trust that consistent effort will produce solid results.

Chapter 15: Speaking Clearly and Listening Well

Good communication can open many doors in life after prison. When you speak in a calm, clear way, people tend to respect and trust you more. When you learn to listen well, you avoid misunderstandings and show others that you value their thoughts. Whether you are trying to explain your skills in a job interview, mend relationships with loved ones, or manage daily conflicts, better speaking and listening skills can bring real benefits.

In this chapter, we explore how to share your ideas more effectively, handle tough conversations, and develop the kind of listening that makes people feel heard. We also look at ways to control anger or frustration when words become heated, and how to say what you need without pushing others away.

---

1. Why Communication Matters After Prison

Once you are out of prison, you may face situations where people judge you or doubt your intentions. Your way of speaking can either confirm their bias or change their view. If you speak aggressively or mumble in a way they cannot follow, they might assume you are rude or hiding something. If you speak politely and clearly, they might see you as someone who is trying to do better.

On the listening side, you might have a lot of stories to tell about what happened, or regrets you feel inside. But if you never pause to hear what others say, you could miss helpful advice or signals. Good communication is a two-way path: you speak with honesty, and you also open up your ears to what the other person brings.

---

2. Checking the Basics of Speaking

Speaking clearly does not mean using fancy words. It means expressing thoughts in a direct, understandable way. Some tips:

1. **Speak at a Steady Pace**
    - Do not rush all your words together. When you speak too fast, people struggle to keep up.

- Also, do not speak so slowly that people get impatient. Aim for a normal, calm pace.

2. **Use Simple Words**
   - Complicated terms can confuse your listener. Pick everyday words.
   - If you are talking about a specialized area—like a certain trade skill—explain it in basic terms if the person seems unfamiliar.

3. **Be Aware of Your Tone**
   - A harsh or mocking tone can offend others, even if your words are not rude.
   - A calm, neutral tone usually helps people listen better, especially when discussing a serious issue.

4. **Keep Eye Contact (if Culturally Appropriate)**
   - Looking someone in the eyes (or near their eye level) shows confidence and honesty.
   - If you constantly look away, they might think you are hiding something.

5. **Mind Your Volume**
   - Speak loud enough to be heard, but not so loud that people feel attacked.

---

3. Overcoming the Fear of Talking

It is normal to feel uneasy when speaking to certain people—like a boss, a landlord, a parole officer, or someone you hurt in the past. Fear can make your voice shake or cause you to forget your words. Some methods to reduce fear:

- **Preparation**: Think about key points before the talk. If needed, jot them on a small card so you do not freeze up.
- **Practice**: Rehearse with a friend or mentor. Even talking in front of a mirror can help.
- **Breathe Steadily**: Before you begin, take a slow, deep breath to calm your nerves.
- **Start with Small Chats**: If you are shy, build confidence by speaking more in low-stakes situations—like casual chats at a community center or volunteer group.

Over time, your anxiety about talking can lessen, especially if you see positive results. When you see people respond well, you gain confidence for the next conversation.

---

4. Explaining Your Situation Without Oversharing

Sometimes you need to mention your criminal record or past troubles in conversation—like in a job interview or a family gathering. You should be honest, but you do not have to give every detail:

1. **Keep It Brief**
    - Summarize the main point. For example, "I was incarcerated due to a bad choice. I have worked hard to learn from it and move forward."
2. **Shift to Growth**
    - Emphasize what you learned, how you have changed, or the steps you are taking to live differently.
3. **Answer Direct Questions**
    - If someone needs more details, provide them calmly. Avoid defensive or angry tones.
4. **Avoid Excuses**
    - Saying "It was not my fault" or blaming others can make you look unwilling to accept responsibility. Acknowledge your role, then show how you are improving.

Sharing just enough builds trust without dragging you into a long, uncomfortable story. It also shows you respect the other person's time and can handle the topic in a mature way.

---

5. Avoiding Slang and Aggressive Language

Prison might have exposed you to slang or aggressive styles of speech. In the outside world, that might cause misunderstandings or push people away. While it is okay to be yourself, you might find it helpful to adjust:

- **Reduce Strong Slang**: If a potential employer or a community program leader cannot understand your slang, they might dismiss you. Practice using words that the general public understands.

- **Limit Swearing**: Some folks take offense easily to curse words, especially in professional settings. Work on replacing curses with calmer expressions.
- **Watch Out for Threatening Expressions**: Phrases like "I'm gonna teach him a lesson" or "He's gonna regret that" can raise red flags. If you are upset, say, "I'm frustrated," or "I don't appreciate that," rather than making it sound like a threat.

Speaking in a balanced way can help you adapt to different environments: job interviews, social events, or even legal appointments. You can still keep a personal style but learn when and where certain words might harm your chances.

---

6. The Art of Listening

Talking is only half of communication. The other half—listening—is often neglected. Good listening helps you learn, solve problems, and build better relationships. Some listening tips:

1. **Pay Full Attention**
   - Put away your phone, turn off the TV, or pause what you are doing. Look at the speaker.
2. **Do Not Interrupt**
   - Let them finish their idea before you chime in. Interruptions can make them feel disrespected.
3. **Use Simple Responses**
   - Nod, say "I see," or "That makes sense." This shows you are following along.
4. **Ask Follow-Up Questions**
   - If something is not clear, ask politely. "Can you explain a bit more about that?" or "What do you mean by...?"
5. **Summarize What You Heard**
   - When they are done, restate the main point: "So you are saying...?" This confirms you understood.

Many disagreements come from poor listening. By focusing on the other person's words, you reduce the chance of jumping to the wrong conclusion.

7. Handling Heated Conversations

In prison, conflicts might have escalated quickly for self-defense or to stand your ground. Outside, lashing out can cost you a job, a home, or your freedom. Here is how to manage heated talks:

- **Stay Calm in Tone**: Lower your volume if the other person is yelling. Often, they will match your level over time.
- **Acknowledge Feelings**: If someone is upset, say, "I hear you're angry. Let's see how we can fix this." This step can defuse tension because they feel understood.
- **Propose a Solution**: Instead of blaming, offer ways to solve the problem: "How about we try...?" or "Would it help if I...?"
- **Know When to Pause**: If the conversation is getting out of control, it is okay to say, "Let's take a break and talk later." Walking away calmly is better than yelling.

Your aim is not to let people walk all over you, but to guide the talk toward a solution. Remember that reactivity can lead to trouble, especially if you are still on parole or trying to maintain a good record.

---

8. Speaking in Job Interviews or Official Meetings

You may face interviews with employers or have meetings with parole officers, social workers, or landlords. A good approach:

1. **Prepare Talking Points**
    - Know what key topics you need to address: your strengths, any qualifications, how you plan to stay on track, etc.
2. **Be Concise**
    - Officials and employers have limited time. Make your points clearly and avoid rambling.
3. **Show Respect**
    - Use polite language: "Yes, sir/ma'am," or "Thank you for your time." Keep a calm posture.
4. **Highlight Improvements**
    - If you have taken classes or earned certificates, mention them briefly to show you are serious.
5. **Ask Relevant Questions**

- At the end, you might ask, "Is there anything else you would like to know about my background?" or "Could you explain the next step?"

Presenting yourself well increases your odds of a positive outcome, whether it is a job offer or a parole meeting that goes smoothly.

---

9. Apologizing and Repairing Damage Through Words

After prison, you might need to apologize to people you hurt or disappointed. A real apology includes:

1. **Taking Responsibility**
   - Admit what you did without blaming others. "I made a bad choice that harmed you."
2. **Expressing Regret**
   - Show that you understand their pain: "I'm sorry for what I put you through."
3. **Explaining Changes**
   - Mention what you are doing to avoid repeating the mistake: "I've been going to counseling and have learned better ways to deal with stress."
4. **Offering to Make Amends**
   - If possible, ask if there is something you can do to ease their hurt or rebuild trust.

Do not expect instant forgiveness. Some might reject your apology or need time. That is their right. Your job is to show genuine remorse and a willingness to do better moving forward.

---

10. Setting Verbal Boundaries

Not every conversation is safe or healthy. Sometimes you need to protect yourself from harmful words or topics:

- **Say "No" Firmly**
  - If someone tries to draw you into illegal schemes or nasty gossip, state clearly: "I'm not interested. Let's change the subject."

- **Refuse Harmful Discussions**
    - If a topic triggers anger or shame and the person keeps pushing, say, "I'm not comfortable talking about this right now."
- **Walk Away if Needed**
    - You do not have to stand there while someone verbally abuses you. Remove yourself and explain calmly that you will return to the discussion when both sides can be respectful.

Boundaries are not about being rude. They protect your mental well-being and help you avoid trouble.

---

11. Building Confidence in Your Voice

If you spent years not speaking up or expressing yourself only through anger, building a new voice takes practice. Some steps to gain confidence:

1. **Record Yourself**
    - Use a phone or any device to record a short message. Listen to your tone, speed, and clarity. Identify areas to improve, like speaking too fast or trailing off at the end of sentences.
2. **Join Toastmasters or a Local Speaking Group**
    - If available, these groups teach public speaking in a supportive environment. It might feel scary at first, but it can accelerate your skills.
3. **Read Aloud**
    - Pick a short article or passage from a book and read it out loud daily. This trains your mouth and tongue to form words clearly.
4. **Get Feedback**
    - Ask a trusted friend or mentor to point out habits that might be distracting—like using filler words ("um," "like") too often.

The more you practice, the more natural it becomes. It might feel strange at first, especially if you have never focused on communication skills, but each attempt helps.

---

12. Listening to Improve Relationships

Communication is the glue of relationships. If you have strained ties with family, children, or old friends, better listening can mend some of the damage:

- **Create a Safe Space**
    - Tell them, "I want to hear how you feel. You can speak freely, and I'll listen without judging."
- **Avoid Defending Too Quickly**
    - Even if they blame you, hold off on defending yourself right away. Let them finish. Then calmly share your perspective.
- **Show Empathy**
    - Say things like, "I see how that could hurt you," or "I get why you are upset." This does not mean you agree with everything; it shows you understand their feelings.
- **Agree on Action**
    - If the goal is to fix something, ask, "What can we both do to make this better?" Turn it into a plan, not just talk.

Better listening does not guarantee people will forgive or trust you instantly, but it lays a groundwork that might lead to healthier bonds over time.

---

13. Dealing with Confusion and Asking Clarifying Questions

You might face situations where someone uses unfamiliar terms or talks about a process you do not understand. Rather than pretend you know, speak up:

- **Admit It**
    - Say, "I'm not sure I follow. Can you explain that part again?"
- **Request Examples**
    - "Could you give me a quick example of what you mean?"
- **Paraphrase**
    - "So if I understand right, you're saying _____."
- **Stay Polite**
    - Asking questions is not a sign of stupidity. It shows you want to avoid mistakes or misunderstandings.

People often appreciate when you clarify rather than guess and create confusion. This is true in work, legal matters, or personal conversations.

---

14. Small Talk and Social Skills

Not all communication is serious or about conflict. Building small talk skills can help you fit into everyday life—like chatting with coworkers or neighbors. Tips for small talk:

1. **Ask Simple Questions**
   - "How's your day going?" or "Did you watch that game last night?"
2. **Find Common Ground**
   - If they mention an interest you share, say, "I like that too. Let's talk more about it."
3. **Keep It Light**
   - Avoid heavy topics like politics or personal trauma in casual chats.
4. **Use Friendly Body Language**
   - Smile if appropriate, nod to show interest, keep a relaxed stance.

Small talk might seem pointless, but it helps build rapport. People tend to open up more deeply when they trust you in simple day-to-day chats first.

---

15. Turning Conflicts into Problem-Solving

Sometimes, a conversation starts calmly but moves toward disagreement. Instead of letting it become a full fight, steer it into problem-solving:

- **Identify the Core Problem**
  - "It sounds like the real issue is we have different views on how to handle money."
- **Suggest Brainstorming**
  - "Let's list possible solutions without judging them yet. Then we can pick what works best."
- **Stay on One Topic**
  - Avoid bringing up old grudges or unrelated issues. Stick to the current conflict.
- **Agree on Next Steps**
  - End by deciding who will do what, and by when. This ensures the talk leads to action, not just venting.

When you approach conflicts this way, you show maturity and reduce the chance of escalation that can harm relationships or get you in trouble.

---

16. Handling Communication on Social Media or Text

In modern life, much communication happens through texts, social media, or email. Words can be easily misunderstood there, because people cannot see your face or hear your tone:

- **Watch Your Tone**
    - If you are upset, your words can read as harsh. Re-read before sending to ensure it does not sound more aggressive than you intend.
- **Keep It Simple**
    - Long paragraphs can confuse readers. If it is a big topic, maybe talk in person or by phone instead.
- **Avoid Argument Spirals**
    - Online fights can get out of hand. If someone provokes you, step back. You do not have to engage in every rude comment.
- **Be Mindful of Privacy**
    - If you are sharing personal stories, remember that screens can be saved or forwarded. Do not post sensitive things publicly if you might regret them later.

Proper online communication is especially important if you are job searching or connecting with professionals. Employers often check social media, so keep your public image respectful.

---

17. Learning from Communication Mistakes

Nobody is perfect at communication, especially if prison life shaped your ways of talking. You might slip up—yell, swear, or shut someone down by accident. When that happens:

- **Own the Error**
    - "I'm sorry for shouting earlier. That was not the right way to speak."
- **Reflect on Why**
    - Were you stressed, hungry, or triggered by a certain topic? Knowing the cause can help you prevent repeats.
- **Plan a Better Response**
    - Next time you feel that anger building, you might use a deep breathing technique or ask to pause the talk.
- **Move Forward**
    - Do not dwell on the mistake too long. Use it as a lesson to refine your approach.

This growth mindset transforms slip-ups into opportunities to improve.

18. Practicing Empathy

Empathy means imagining what the other person might be feeling. When you empathize, you speak in a kinder way and understand deeper reasons behind someone's words:

- **Look Beyond the Words**
    - If someone is shouting, they might be scared or hurt underneath. Try to see that instead of just hearing the anger.
- **Use Empathy Statements**
    - "I see this is really important to you," or "I can tell this worries you a lot."
- **Ask About Their View**
    - "How does this situation make you feel?" Then give them time to answer.

Empathy reduces friction. Even if you disagree with someone's view, acknowledging their feelings often leads to a calmer, more productive talk.

---

19. Building a Personal Communication Plan

If you know you have certain weaknesses—like interrupting, cursing, or shutting down when criticized—you can create a plan to improve. It might include:

1. **A Daily Reminder**
    - Write a note: "Speak calmly. Listen fully. Ask questions." Read it each morning.
2. **Specific Goals**
    - For example, "Today, I will not interrupt anyone at work," or "I will use zero curse words during this family visit."
3. **Check-In with a Friend**
    - Ask a trusted mentor to ask you once a week how you are doing with your communication goals.
4. **Celebrate Small Steps**
    - If you go a full day without snapping at someone, recognize that progress.

A structured approach can help you form new habits faster than just hoping it happens.

20. Conclusion of Chapter 15

Speaking clearly and listening well may seem like simple acts, but they are powerful tools for building a stable life after prison. By choosing your words carefully, using a respectful tone, and showing others you value their views, you open doors that might have stayed locked otherwise—jobs, healthier relationships, and less conflict overall.

True communication is a mix of both honesty and empathy. You share what is on your mind in a calm, direct way, and you also make space to hear what others need to say. This balance can repair old wounds, prevent new fights, and show that you have grown beyond the person you were when you first entered the prison gates.

These skills are not learned in a day. You will likely make mistakes, raise your voice, or fail to listen sometimes. But each conversation is a new chance to practice. Keep working on your clarity, your tone, and your listening. Over time, you will see that strong communication not only helps you stay out of trouble but also helps you create a more positive, respectful circle around you—whether that is at work, at home, or among neighbors and friends.

Chapter 16: Finding Purpose in the Middle of Challenges

Life after prison can feel like climbing a steep hill. You might struggle with past regrets, face legal obstacles, and worry about how others see you. In the midst of these pressures, finding a sense of purpose can keep you from giving up. Purpose does not mean you have to join a grand mission. It is about having a deeper reason for your daily actions, something that sparks motivation and keeps you focused on what truly matters.

In this chapter, we explore how to find or create purpose even in tough circumstances. We look at how small daily choices link to bigger meanings, how to use your strengths to serve goals beyond yourself, and how to keep going when setbacks appear. Whether your purpose is linked to family, faith, personal growth, or making a positive mark on your community, it can become a guiding force that helps you stay on a steady path.

---

1. What "Purpose" Really Means

Purpose is the sense that your life has direction and that you matter in the world around you. It is not just a job title or a big dream. It is the core reason you get up each morning. A few examples:

- **Being a Good Father or Mentor**: Some men find purpose in guiding their children or helping younger relatives avoid bad choices.
- **Improving the Community**: Others volunteer or work to make their neighborhood safer or more welcoming.
- **Growing in Faith**: For some, spiritual or religious commitments bring meaning.
- **Pursuing Skills and Knowledge**: Some discover purpose by mastering a trade or subject, using it to uplift themselves and others.

Your purpose should match your values and experiences. It is unique to you. Even if it starts as a small spark, it can grow into a steady light that keeps you focused when life feels stormy.

---

2. Why Purpose Matters After Prison

Without a sense of purpose, it is easy to drift or return to old habits. Stress, temptation, and doubts can drag you down if you do not have something bigger to aim for. Purposeful living helps in several ways:

- **Stronger Resilience**: You bounce back more easily after failure because you see the bigger picture.
- **Less Temptation**: You have a reason not to slip into crime or substance abuse. Breaking your purpose is harder than breaking a simple rule.
- **Clarity in Choices**: Decisions become easier because you weigh them against your purpose. If your purpose is to support your family, you will be less likely to gamble your paycheck or hang out with the wrong crowd.
- **Fulfillment**: Knowing you are moving toward something meaningful can give you joy, even when you face difficulties.

Purpose does not erase your problems, but it gives you a positive direction to move forward.

---

3. Reflecting on Your Past to Shape Purpose

Your past mistakes, regrets, and even your prison experience can hold clues to your purpose. Ask yourself:

1. **What Did I Learn in Prison?**
   - Did you discover any skills, insights, or new viewpoints? Maybe you realized you enjoy teaching others, or you found out you are good at a certain trade.
2. **What Do I Regret Most?**
   - Regret might point you to a purpose, such as making amends or preventing others from doing what you did.
3. **Which Parts of My Old Life Do I Want to Leave Behind?**
   - That could mean cutting ties with crime, a gang, or a mindset of hopelessness.
4. **What Am I Proud Of?**
   - Even in prison, you might have moments of helping someone, learning something, or showing discipline. Those can hint at possible paths forward.

Turning negative experiences into a lesson can feed a stronger purpose. It does not mean ignoring the harm done—it means using what you learned to live more meaningfully now.

4. Finding What Sparks You

If you are not sure what your deeper purpose is, try exploring new activities or reflecting on what makes you feel alive:

- **Try Different Volunteer Work**
    - Helping at a local food bank or community center might show you a cause that resonates.
- **Read or Watch Inspiring Stories**
    - Learn about people who overcame hardships and see if anything they did connects with you.
- **Speak to Mentors or Community Leaders**
    - Ask what drives them. Sometimes hearing about their purpose can spark ideas in you.
- **Note Small Joys**
    - Pay attention to daily moments that make you feel good—like fixing something, offering advice, or comforting someone. Those clues might point to a bigger sense of mission.

Finding purpose is not always dramatic. It often grows from small hints and repeated interests.

5. Setting Goals Linked to Purpose

Once you sense what matters to you, link that to concrete goals (see Chapter 14). For example:

- If your purpose is **being a supportive father**, you might set a goal to spend quality time with your child daily, attend parent-teacher meetings, or improve your income so you can provide more.
- If your purpose is **helping others avoid crime**, you might aim to speak at a local youth center or join an outreach program that mentors at-risk teens.

- If your purpose is **spiritual growth**, you might plan to read spiritual texts regularly, attend services, or join a study group.

Goals turn abstract ideas into real steps you can take. They make your purpose concrete.

---

6. Balancing Personal Gain and Service to Others

Purpose often includes bettering yourself and helping others. If you only focus on yourself, you might feel lonely or miss the power of serving people around you. If you only give to others but neglect your own stability, you might burn out. Find a balance:

- **Improve Yourself**
    - Work on your health, finances, and mindset so you are strong enough to help.
- **Give Back**
    - Use your time, skills, or even small donations if you can, to support causes you care about.
- **Share Knowledge**
    - If you learned something valuable—like how to handle anger—consider guiding someone else who struggles.

This blend can keep you growing while also strengthening the community or family around you.

---

7. Overcoming Doubts About Worthiness

A common barrier is feeling unworthy of a good purpose. You might think, "Who am I to aim for something high after all I have done?" That mindset can trap you in shame and hold you back. Recognize that:

- **Past Mistakes Do Not Erase Future Possibilities**
    - Many people who caused harm later dedicated themselves to positive work.
- **Change Is Possible**
    - If you are making an honest effort, you have every right to pursue a meaningful path.

- **Others Have Forgiven and Moved On**
    - You might be the only one clinging to the idea that you are not worthy.

Give yourself permission to aim for a purpose. Doubts will come, but they do not have to define your path.

---

8. Dealing with Setbacks

Having a purpose does not mean everything falls into place easily. You may still lose a job, face family conflicts, or struggle with health. Setbacks happen. The difference is how you handle them:

- **Remember Your Why**
    - Reconnect with the deeper reason you got started. This can keep you from quitting when you stumble.
- **Adjust If Needed**
    - Maybe you need to shift your focus temporarily. For instance, if you get injured, you cannot volunteer physically, but you might help with phone calls or planning.
- **Seek Help**
    - Talk to mentors, counselors, or friends. Let them remind you of your progress and the bigger picture.

Each hurdle, when overcome, makes your purpose stronger. You prove to yourself that you will not back down when life tests you.

---

9. Tying Purpose to Your Daily Routine

Purpose is not just for big moments. It is woven into everyday actions. Examples:

- **Morning Check-In**
    - Remind yourself why you are getting up and what you plan to achieve. One or two sentences can set the tone.
- **Meaningful Work Approach**
    - Even if your job is simple or not glamorous, do it with care because it supports your bigger goals—like financial stability or caring for your family.

- **Treating People Kindly**
    - If part of your purpose is to spread positivity or help others, reflect that in how you treat coworkers, neighbors, and strangers.
- **Bedtime Reflection**
    - Ask, "Did I live closer to my purpose today? Where can I improve tomorrow?"

These small touches keep you focused on purpose, not just survival.

---

10. Using Past Hurts to Connect with Others

If your purpose involves helping people who face issues similar to yours, your own scars can become part of your strength. For example:

- **Speaking at Recovery Groups**
    - If you beat an addiction, your story might inspire others.
- **Helping At-Risk Youth**
    - Teens might listen to you more if they know you have real-life experience with crime or gang life.
- **Supporting Families of Inmates**
    - You might understand their concerns better than someone who has never been involved with the prison system.

Your pain can become a bridge to empathy. Of course, do not push your story on people who are not ready to hear it, but do not hide it if it can offer hope.

---

11. Finding Role Models of Purpose

Look for examples of people who found purpose after major challenges—could be local folks you know or famous individuals:

- **Neighbors or Community Leaders**
    - Some might have been in prison and turned their lives around. Learn how they found their purpose.
- **Biographies or Documentaries**
    - Reading or watching stories about people who overcame struggles can spark ideas for your own life.
- **Online Communities**

- If you have internet access, you can find stories of reentry success. But be careful to follow legitimate sources, not fake claims.

You do not need to copy someone's path. Just let their stories remind you that it is never too late to do meaningful things.

---

12. Checking Your Inner Values

Purpose aligns closely with values—the things you deeply care about. If you are unsure of your values, consider:

- **Justice**: Do you believe in fairness and want to correct wrongs?
- **Family**: Is being a reliable partner, parent, or sibling your top priority?
- **Faith or Spiritual Growth**: Do spiritual practices guide your moral compass?
- **Education or Skill-Building**: Do you value learning and becoming an expert at something?
- **Community Care**: Do you want to protect or improve the place where you live?

Once you see your core values, you can shape a purpose that respects them.

---

13. Coping with Critics and Naysayers

Not everyone will support your new sense of purpose. Some might doubt you, bring up your past, or say you will never change. A few ways to handle this:

- **Focus on Honest Action**
    - Over time, consistent action speaks louder than words. If you keep living your purpose, some critics might soften.
- **Limit Contact**
    - If certain people only tear you down, reduce how often you see them, especially if they threaten your resolve.
- **Stay Calm**
    - Avoid shouting matches. A short, polite response like "I understand you feel that way, but I'm working to live differently" might be enough. Then keep doing what you know is right.

Your purpose is personal. You do not need everyone's approval to follow it. Surround yourself with those who encourage positive growth.

---

14. Renewing Purpose Over Time

Purposes can evolve. What drives you in your first year out of prison may change later. Maybe at first, your main purpose is to stabilize your life and stay free. Once you reach stability, you might yearn to do more—like starting a small business or guiding youth. It is okay to refine your purpose as you learn and grow:

- **Review Every So Often**
    - Ask, "Is this purpose still what drives me?" If yes, keep going. If no, adjust.
- **Add New Goals**
    - As you succeed in certain areas, set fresh goals that reflect your growth.
- **Stay Open**
    - Sometimes unexpected events spark a new direction, like a volunteer project that becomes your true calling.

Change can be a sign of progress, not confusion, as long as you remain honest with yourself about where your heart leads.

---

15. Handling Low Points

Even with purpose, you will have low days—moments of depression, high stress, or feeling alone. Some ways to get through them:

- **Lean on Support**
    - Call a friend, counselor, or join a support group. Tell them you are struggling.
- **Do Something Small That Connects to Your Purpose**
    - Even a tiny step, like reading an inspirational paragraph or doing a small good deed, can remind you of your bigger reason.
- **Allow Yourself to Feel**

- Suppressing sadness or anger can make things worse. Let it out in healthy ways, like writing or talking to a therapist, then refocus on your goals.
- **Remember Past Victories**
    - You have overcome obstacles before—like surviving prison or beating a tough habit. That strength is still inside you.

Low points do not mean your purpose is gone. They are challenges to reaffirm why you chose this path in the first place.

---

16. Celebrating (Marking) Achievements Linked to Purpose

As you move along, recognize important progress toward your purpose:

- **Note Personal Milestones**
    - If your purpose is to be a steady father, mark the day you started consistently helping your child with homework.
- **Share with Trusted People**
    - If you volunteer regularly, mention how it makes you feel to a friend or mentor. Hearing their support can boost your motivation.
- **Reflect in a Journal**
    - Write down how you felt when you took a meaningful step. This record becomes a source of encouragement later.

---

17. Turning Purpose into a Legacy

Think about what you want to leave behind, even in small ways:

- **Family Legacy**
    - Teach your kids lessons you learned the hard way so they do not repeat them.
- **Community Legacy**
    - Improve your block or your neighborhood in some practical manner—like organizing cleanups or mentoring younger neighbors.
- **Workplace Legacy**
    - If you are known for reliability and helpfulness at your job, that leaves a good mark on coworkers who meet you.

You do not need to be famous or wealthy to have a legacy. Every bit of good you do can ripple outward, especially if you remain consistent.

---

18. Avoiding Purpose Burnout

Sometimes people get so fired up about a cause that they neglect their own needs, leading to exhaustion. Balance is vital:

- **Schedule Down Time**
    - Even if you have big goals, take a day or an afternoon each week to rest or do something relaxing.
- **Ask for Help**
    - Delegate tasks if you are part of a group project. You do not have to carry everything alone.
- **Maintain Health and Finances**
    - Your purpose might be community work, but you still need to pay your bills and keep yourself healthy.

Burnout can sour your view of your purpose. Keep your physical, mental, and emotional well-being in mind, so you can stay strong in the long run.

---

19. Examples of Small Daily Purposes

Purpose does not always have to be grand. Here are smaller, day-to-day examples that add up:

- **Being Kind to One Person Each Day**
    - Even if it is just a friendly greeting or a small help.
- **Learning One New Skill Per Month**
    - This can range from cooking a healthy meal to fixing a simple house problem.
- **Spending Quiet Time for Self-Reflection**
    - Maybe 10 minutes of sitting in silence or writing down gratitude points.
- **Keeping Promises**
    - Each time you do what you said you would, you build your sense of integrity.

When you link these small habits to your overall purpose (like "I'm learning new skills so I can find better work and support my family"), they become meaningful building blocks.

---

20. Conclusion of Chapter 16

Finding or creating purpose after prison can change your life's direction. It gives you a reason to face each day with determination, even when challenges feel heavy. Your purpose does not need to be flashy or recognized by everyone. It just has to be real for you—something that resonates with your values, uses your strengths, and pushes you to grow beyond past mistakes.

By reflecting on your experiences, identifying what truly matters to you, and setting goals in line with that deeper sense of direction, you build a path that goes beyond mere survival. You become someone who strives for something better—for yourself, your loved ones, and possibly your community.

Expect obstacles and doubt. You will stumble, question your worth, and face critics. But purpose is what keeps you getting back up. It anchors you in the belief that you can make a positive mark, no matter where you have been. Whether your purpose is about family, personal growth, faith, or helping those who might fall into the traps you once knew, let it guide your actions daily. Over time, you will see that living with purpose can shape not only your future but also bring new strength to your everyday life.

Chapter 17: Improving Your Self-Worth

Self-worth is the belief that you have value as a person. It goes deeper than feeling confident about a skill or being proud of an achievement. It is about seeing yourself as someone who deserves respect and good things in life, regardless of past mistakes. When men come out of prison, self-worth is often low because of shame, guilt, or negative labels from others. But rebuilding it is possible—and important—because a healthy sense of self-worth can guide you away from bad influences and help you aim for better goals.

This chapter explores the steps you can take to improve how you see yourself, why self-worth matters in day-to-day life, and how to protect it when challenges arise. As you discover more reasons to appreciate yourself, you will find it easier to stay on track and treat yourself and others with more kindness.

---

1. What Self-Worth Really Means

Self-worth is not about bragging or feeling "better" than other people. Instead, it is a steady sense that you, as a human being, have value. You recognize that your life matters, your feelings matter, and your growth matters. This does not mean you ignore your faults or your past. It means you refuse to define yourself only by your errors or by negative judgments from others.

Some signs of healthy self-worth include:

- Believing you deserve a second chance.
- Treating your body and mind with respect.
- Standing up for yourself in a calm way when people mistreat you.
- Knowing you can learn from mistakes rather than letting them crush your spirit.

It helps to see self-worth as an ongoing relationship with yourself. You may have good days when you feel strong and days when you doubt yourself. The goal is to keep building positive habits that support a kinder view of who you are.

---

2. Why Low Self-Worth Is Common After Prison

Time behind bars can shape how you view yourself. You might feel shame for the crime, guilt for hurting people, or anger at the system. You may have lost jobs, relationships, or personal freedoms. People in your life might remind you of your mistakes or treat you as if you have no worth. All of this can push your self-worth down.

Also, prisons often demand that you appear tough on the outside. You cannot show weakness or you risk being taken advantage of. After release, you might have trouble shifting from that hard shell to a healthier sense of self. Or you might have internalized negative labels, telling yourself, "I am just a criminal."

Recognizing these factors helps you understand why you feel the way you do. It also reminds you that these feelings are normal, not proof that you truly lack worth. They are a result of your experiences, and experiences can be moved past with effort.

---

3. Identifying Negative Self-Talk

Negative self-talk is the unkind voice in your head that says things like:

- "You are too messed up to change."
- "Nobody will ever trust you again."
- "You will fail anyway, so why try?"

These thoughts often pop up automatically, without you realizing it. Over time, they damage your self-worth, making you believe you cannot improve. The first step to dealing with negative self-talk is to notice when it happens. Pay attention to moments when you feel a sharp drop in mood or confidence—often, a negative thought triggered that feeling.

Once you catch these thoughts, challenge them. Ask yourself: "Is this really true, or is this my shame or fear talking?" For example, if your mind says, "I will fail anyway," remind yourself of a time you succeeded at something—even a small success like completing a prison course, resolving a conflict peacefully, or keeping a promise to someone.

---

4. Replacing Negative Thoughts with Balanced Ones

You do not have to become unrealistically positive, but you can adopt more balanced self-talk, such as:

- "I made mistakes, but I am working hard to change."
- "Some people may reject me, but not everyone."
- "I can learn new skills if I put in the effort."

When you notice a negative thought like "I will never get a job," replace it with something like "Many people with records do find work, and I can improve my chances by preparing well."

This simple switch is powerful. At first, it might feel forced, but over time, it teaches your mind to look for possibilities instead of shutting down.

---

5. Treating Yourself with Respect

Improving self-worth means taking actions that show you respect yourself. That can include:

1. **Caring for Your Body**
    - Eating healthy meals, getting regular sleep, and doing basic exercise. Even small steps—like walking more or cutting back on junk food—signal that you see your body as valuable.
2. **Setting Boundaries**
    - If someone constantly puts you down, it is okay to limit contact or speak up about how they treat you. Respecting yourself means not letting others harm your well-being.
3. **Avoiding Self-Punishment**
    - If you slip up on a goal or face a setback, do not beat yourself up for days. Learn from it and move forward.
4. **Seeking Support**
    - Seeing a counselor or joining a support group is a sign of strength and self-care. It shows you believe you are worth the effort to heal and grow.

When you act like a person who deserves decent treatment, your brain starts believing it more and more.

6. Building on Strengths

Everyone has strengths, even if you do not see them immediately. Maybe you are good with your hands, or you have a knack for calming people down, or you are disciplined in a certain routine. Identifying and using these strengths can boost your self-worth. Some ways to do this:

- **Make a List of Skills**
    - Think about what you can do well, whether it is fixing cars, cooking basic meals, or organizing tasks. Write them down.
- **Use Them Often**
    - If you are good at repairing things, offer to help a neighbor with a minor fix. If you have a calming presence, support a friend who is stressed.
- **Learn New Skills**
    - Expanding your skill set also expands your self-worth. Each time you learn something new, you prove you are capable.

Seeing yourself succeed, even in small tasks, forms a healthier view of your abilities and potential.

7. Avoiding Comparisons to Others

You might see people around you who never went to prison and feel jealous or ashamed. Or you might see someone with a record who has already built a great life outside and wonder why you are behind. These comparisons can damage self-worth. Remember:

- **Everyone Has Different Starting Points**
    - Some folks had strong family support or better opportunities. Others had more struggles. Your path is your own.
- **Progress Over Perfection**
    - Aim to improve from where you were yesterday, not to match someone else's life.
- **Learn from Others Without Feeling Inferior**
    - If you see someone who overcame hurdles, get inspired or ask them for tips, rather than feeling worthless in comparison.

Comparisons often ignore the hidden battles people face. Focus on your journey and celebrate each step (or "mark" each step) forward without putting yourself down.

---

8. Setting Achievable Challenges

Challenging yourself can increase self-worth. It shows you can handle adversity and grow. The key is to set challenges that are tough enough to stretch you but not so hard that you give up. For instance:

- **Physical Challenges**
    - Maybe you aim to walk or jog a certain distance each week.
- **Learning Challenges**
    - You could decide to improve reading skills, learn computer basics, or master a trade.
- **Social Challenges**
    - If you tend to avoid people, challenge yourself to speak to one new person a week or to participate in a group activity.

Each time you complete a challenge, your sense of "I can do this" grows. Be patient if you fail or need extra tries—it is part of learning.

---

9. Recognizing Progress Over Time

Self-worth grows when you notice your gains, no matter how small. Keep track in a notebook or on your phone:

- **Daily or Weekly Wins**
    - For example, "I stayed calm in a conflict" or "I managed my money better this week."
- **Monthly Reflections**
    - Look back and see how you have improved. Maybe a month ago, you felt hopeless, but now you have a part-time job or a more positive mindset.
- **Longer-Term Changes**
    - After six months or a year, note big changes, like paying off a debt or rebuilding a family relationship.

Progress can feel slow, but these written records remind you that you are indeed moving forward.

---

10. Dealing with Criticism

At times, people might criticize you because of your past or how you act now. Some criticism might be valid and helpful, while other criticism is just harsh or mean. You can handle it by:

1. **Listening for Truth**
   - Is there a real point in their words that can help you improve? If so, consider it. If not, let it go.
2. **Avoid Getting Defensive**
   - Angrily lashing back often confirms their negative view. Respond calmly or walk away if they are being cruel without reason.
3. **Setting Boundaries**
   - If someone repeatedly insults you, limit contact or tell them firmly that you will not engage with disrespect.

Healthy self-worth means you can take constructive feedback without crumbling, and you can reject unfair attacks without internalizing them.

---

11. Surrounding Yourself with Positive Influences

People around you have a strong impact on how you see yourself. Try to spend more time with those who:

- Encourage you to do better.
- Acknowledge your efforts.
- Give honest feedback kindly.
- Respect your boundaries.

Avoid or reduce contact with people who constantly drag you down or tempt you into negative behaviors. Even if you cannot cut them out entirely (like certain family members), you can limit how often you see them or steer the conversation away from harmful topics. A supportive community can lift your self-worth by reminding you of your strengths and goals.

12. Giving to Others as a Self-Worth Booster

Sometimes, doing good for others can raise your sense of value. This does not mean ignoring your own needs, but small acts of kindness can make you feel useful. For example:

- **Helping a Neighbor**
    - If you have a skill—like fixing a leaky faucet—offer to help someone who needs it.
- **Volunteering**
    - Join a local event, a church group, or a reentry program that helps others.
- **Sharing Your Experience**
    - If you have learned lessons in prison or during recovery, talk to younger people who might be heading down the wrong path.

When you see that your actions can lighten someone else's load, you realize you are capable of bringing positive change. That is a huge boost to self-worth.

13. Facing Old Feelings of Guilt or Shame

Sometimes, your sense of low self-worth is tangled in deep guilt for what you did or who you hurt. Dealing with guilt can be a slow process, but it is key to rebuilding self-worth. Steps might include:

- **Accepting Responsibility**
    - Recognize that you caused pain, but do not let that define your entire identity forever.
- **Making Amends** (If Possible)
    - A sincere apology or act of restitution can help you let go of guilt. Some people may not accept it, and that is their choice.
- **Learning from the Mistake**
    - Ask, "What can I learn from this that will help me live differently?" Focus on future actions, not just regrets about the past.
- **Forgiving Yourself**
    - This does not mean excusing the harm done. It means understanding you are more than your worst act, and you are allowed to move forward.

Heavy shame can keep you stuck. Working through it (possibly with a counselor or mentor) frees you to see that you are still worthy of living a decent life.

---

14. Balancing Confidence and Humility

Self-worth does not mean arrogance. You can believe in your value without belittling others or acting like you are always right. A balanced approach:

- **Confidence**: "I can handle challenges and keep growing."
- **Humility**: "I do not know everything, and I can learn from others."

This balance makes you more relatable. People often respect someone who has quiet confidence rather than a loud, boastful attitude.

---

15. Building Self-Worth Through Mindful Choices

Every day, you make dozens of choices—from what time you wake up to how you handle stress. Each choice can either build or harm your self-worth. For example:

- **Choice to Stay Clean**
    - Avoiding drugs or excessive alcohol protects your health and keeps your mind clear.
- **Choice to Show Up on Time**
    - Demonstrates responsibility, which can boost how you see yourself and how others see you.
- **Choice to Communicate Kindly**
    - Using respectful words, even if you are annoyed, helps you feel in control and decent.
- **Choice to Follow Parole Rules**
    - Each time you honor those conditions, you prove to yourself you are disciplined and serious about your new path.

Mindful choices add up. They reinforce a narrative: "I am someone who respects myself and my future."

---

16. Recognizing When You Need Professional Help

Sometimes, deep shame or past trauma might block your self-worth more seriously. If you find yourself stuck in dark moods or self-harming thoughts, consider seeking professional help. Signs include:

- Feeling hopeless all the time.
- Inability to handle day-to-day tasks due to low self-esteem.
- Frequent thoughts of hurting yourself.
- Reliving past trauma intensely, which sabotages your progress.

Counselors or psychologists can guide you through deeper issues. Many communities have free or low-cost services, especially for people reentering society. Getting this help does not mean you are weak. It means you care enough about yourself to heal.

---

17. Practicing Gratitude

Gratitude means noticing and being thankful for what is good in your life. Even if your situation is tough, there are likely small positives—a supportive friend, a safe place to sleep, a skill you have, or simply the fact that you are free from prison. Practicing gratitude helps shift your mindset from "I am lacking" to "I do have some good in my life." Some methods:

- **Daily Gratitude Lists**
    - Write down three things you are thankful for each day.
- **Mentally Revisit Good Moments**
    - Think back on any kind words you received, or small successes you had.
- **Thank People**
    - Telling someone "I appreciate your help" not only makes them feel good; it reminds you that you are cared for.

Gratitude takes focus off your flaws and shows you that despite mistakes, life can still offer things to value.

---

18. Role of Forgiving Others

Holding onto anger or grudges against people who hurt you can feed a cycle of negativity that lowers your self-worth. It keeps you tied to bitterness. Forgiving others (where safe and appropriate) can free you to focus on your own growth. It does not mean letting them off the hook or inviting them back into your life if they are dangerous. It means you choose not to let hate poison you. By letting go of that weight, you can stand a bit taller in your own eyes.

---

19. Creating a Self-Worth Routine

You can form daily or weekly habits that nurture self-worth:

1. **Morning Affirmation**
   - Say a short phrase like, "I am working to be a good person today," or "I am worthy of a fresh start."
2. **Brief Check-In**
   - At midday or bedtime, ask yourself: "Did my actions match the person I want to be?" If not, what can you do tomorrow to improve?
3. **Supportive Reading**
   - Read a quick passage from a book or a motivational quote that reminds you of your value.
4. **Positive Connection**
   - Contact a friend or mentor regularly to exchange supportive words.

Over time, these small routines shift your overall self-image. They keep you from sliding back into self-hate.

---

20. Conclusion of Chapter 17

Improving your self-worth after prison is a key step in forging a stable, honest life. Low self-worth can lead you to sabotage yourself or fall under the influence of people who do not have your best interests at heart. On the other hand, healthy self-worth drives you to aim higher, protect your well-being, and treat others with the respect you want for yourself.

This change does not happen overnight. It involves catching negative self-talk, making better day-to-day choices, and possibly addressing deeper guilt or trauma. Surrounding yourself with supportive influences, building on personal strengths, and recognizing your progress all feed into a stronger sense of self. Even if you stumble, each day is a chance to practice seeing yourself as worthy of better things. By respecting yourself in practical ways—like tending to your health, setting boundaries, and learning new skills—you gradually convince your mind and heart that you do matter. Over time, this healthier self-worth can shape your relationships, your goals, and the entire path you walk after prison.

Chapter 18: Coping with Ups and Downs

Life after prison is rarely a straight line of progress. There will be times when you feel on track—finding a job, reconnecting with family, and staying out of trouble. Then, without warning, you might face a job loss, an argument at home, or legal complications that throw you off balance. Coping with these ups and downs is essential to staying free and building a stable future. It is normal to have good days and bad days, but the key is developing ways to handle the tough moments without giving up or reverting to harmful behaviors.

In this chapter, we explore methods for dealing with both the highs and lows you might experience. We look at how to celebrate small victories (in a modest way) and how to pick yourself up when setbacks threaten to drag you down. By preparing mentally and practically, you can navigate the rollercoaster of life outside prison with greater resilience.

---

1. Understanding the Nature of Ups and Downs

No matter how well you plan, life is unpredictable. You may gain a job one week, then lose it two months later due to layoffs. You might patch things up with a loved one, only to have an old argument flare up. These ups and downs are part of life for everyone, but they can feel more intense when you are also dealing with parole rules, financial stress, or societal judgment.

Learning that highs and lows come and go can help you avoid extremes in your reactions. When something good happens, you can enjoy it without assuming everything will always be perfect. When something bad happens, you can recognize it as a challenge to overcome rather than a sign that you are doomed.

---

2. Marking Small Victories

When you succeed at a task—like finishing a required program, avoiding a tempting situation, or getting positive feedback at work—pause to notice it. You do not have to throw a party, but do acknowledge that you did something right:

- **Write It Down**

- Keep a list of positive outcomes in a small notebook or your phone. Reread them on tough days.
- **Tell a Supporter**
  - Share the news with a friend or mentor who understands your journey. Hearing them say "Well done" can reinforce your sense of progress.
- **Reflect on How You Achieved It**
  - Ask yourself what steps led to the success: "I stayed calm," or "I followed my budget." This helps you see that you can repeat those steps for future successes.

Highlighting these small wins reminds you that, despite setbacks, you are capable of good outcomes. It also helps balance any negative self-talk that tries to overshadow your achievements.

---

3. Expecting and Managing Setbacks

Setbacks do not mean you have failed overall. They are just part of any progress journey. Examples of setbacks might include:

- **Relapsing into Old Habits**
  - You might slip once or twice. Instead of giving up, focus on learning how to prevent the next slip.
- **Financial Problems**
  - A sudden expense or job loss can cripple your budget. You may need to seek temporary help or adjust your plans.
- **Family Tensions**
  - Old wounds can reopen. People may not trust you yet, or they might have their own problems that affect your relationship.

When setbacks happen, remind yourself of the bigger picture. One stumble does not erase the growth you have achieved. Control how you respond: address the immediate issue, seek help if needed, and plan for a better approach next time.

---

4. Staying Grounded During Good Times

Sometimes the biggest risk arises when everything is going well. You might relax your guard, think you no longer need caution, or feel so confident that you take reckless steps. For example:

- **Overconfidence in Finances**
    - If you get a better job or a bonus, you might start overspending, forgetting you still have debts or future needs.
- **Dropping Healthy Routines**
    - Once you feel stable, you might skip support meetings, counseling sessions, or daily check-ins, making it easier for old habits to creep back.
- **Bragging or Provoking Others**
    - Feeling "on top," you might rub it in people's faces, which can lead to conflict.

Keep a humble perspective even in the best times. Appreciate the improvement but stay consistent with the routines and boundaries that got you there. This steadiness protects you from dramatic falls.

---

5. Dealing with Sudden Crises

At some point, you might face a sudden crisis—like a serious health problem, a loved one's crisis, or an unexpected parole violation accusation. Your emotional reaction might be shock or panic. Steps to handle such moments:

1. **Pause and Breathe**
    - Take a few slow breaths to regain some calm before you act.
2. **Assess the Situation**
    - Gather facts: What exactly happened? Who can help? What are the immediate risks?
3. **Reach Out for Support**
    - Call a friend, mentor, or hotline if the crisis is overwhelming. Do not isolate yourself.
4. **Make a Plan**
    - Even a short plan helps you feel more in control. Identify a few steps you can take right away.
5. **Avoid Rash Choices**
    - Resist the urge to do something extreme out of fear or anger—like running away, breaking the law, or burning bridges with loved ones.

This approach does not guarantee an easy fix, but it prevents a crisis from turning into a total spiral.

6. Keeping a Balanced Mindset

When things go well, you might think everything is perfect. When they go poorly, you might feel everything is terrible. A balanced mindset recognizes that reality usually lies somewhere in between. Tips for balance:

- **Identify Gray Areas**
    - Rarely is a situation purely black and white. Maybe you lost your job, but at least you learned some new skills there. Or your family argument was tough, but it also revealed issues you can work on.
- **Use "Yet"**
    - Instead of saying, "I cannot handle this," say, "I cannot handle this yet." That small word keeps the door open for growth.
- **Check the Evidence**
    - If your mind says, "I am a complete failure," list things that prove otherwise: steps you took that show you are trying or areas you have improved.

Balancing your viewpoint prevents emotional whiplash where you over-celebrate the good times and sink into despair during the bad times.

---

7. Creating a Personal Support System for Ups and Downs

No one can handle life's twists alone. Build a network:

- **Friends or Family**
    - Look for people who genuinely care and provide steady encouragement.
- **Support Groups**
    - Reentry groups, substance recovery groups, or faith-based meetings. You share experiences and tips for handling tough situations.
- **Mentors or Counselors**
    - Professionals or volunteers who guide you with more structured help.
- **Online Forums (with Caution)**
    - You might find supportive communities online. Just be careful with sharing personal info and watch for unhelpful or negative discussions.

A good support system can remind you of your goals during your highs and encourage you during your lows. Share both successes and struggles with them. That way, they understand your overall journey and can offer better advice.

---

8. Practical Ways to Adapt When Plans Change

Life will rarely follow your script perfectly. Being flexible can keep you going:

1. **Have a Backup Plan**
   - If Plan A fails, what is Plan B or C? For example, if your job ends, do you have a list of other places to apply or a side gig you can do temporarily?
2. **Remain Calm About Change**
   - Many men panic when routines get disrupted. But change can sometimes lead to better opportunities.
3. **Revisit Your Long-Term Goals**
   - Adjusting daily or weekly plans might be necessary, but keep your eyes on the bigger aims you have (like stable housing, a steady job, or being a good parent).

Adaptation is not about giving up on dreams. It is about finding new routes to reach them when the original path is blocked.

---

9. Using Healthy Coping Skills in Low Times

When you hit a down moment—like feeling depressed, angry, or hopeless—turn to safe coping methods instead of harmful ones (like substance use or violence). Possible safe coping methods:

- **Physical Outlet**
  - Go for a walk, do push-ups, or engage in a simple workout. This can release tension.
- **Writing or Journaling**
  - Putting your feelings on paper can help you process them without acting rashly.
- **Talking**
  - Call a trusted friend or meet a mentor to share what is bothering you.

- **Breathing Exercises**
    - Close your eyes, inhale for four counts, hold for one, exhale for four. Repeat until you feel calmer.
- **Music or Relaxation**
    - Listen to songs that comfort or inspire you, or do a short relaxation exercise.

These methods may not magically fix the problem, but they can steady you enough to think clearly about solutions rather than making things worse.

---

10. Building Emotional Resilience

Emotional resilience means bouncing back when life knocks you down. It is a skill you can strengthen over time by:

- **Learning from Hard Times**
    - Each challenge teaches you something. Maybe you learn a new coping strategy, or you discover who truly has your back.
- **Accepting That Struggle Is Normal**
    - You are not the only one facing hardships. Everyone deals with some form of them. Acknowledging this can reduce self-pity or shame.
- **Maintaining Healthy Habits**
    - A strong body and mind handle stress better. Keep up with sleep, nutrition, and exercise.
- **Keeping Perspective**
    - Remember past troubles you overcame. Those victories show you can do it again.

Resilience is not about never feeling pain; it is about feeling it, dealing with it, and finding a way forward.

---

11. Handling Success Without Sabotage

Some men, after a taste of success, self-sabotage because deep down they do not feel they deserve it or they fear it will not last. Signs of self-sabotage include skipping important meetings, picking fights with helpful people, or suddenly quitting a good job. If you notice these behaviors, ask:

- **Am I Afraid of Failing Eventually?**
    - Sometimes it feels easier to destroy success first than to see it slip away later. Recognize that fear and fight it by reminding yourself you are allowed to succeed.
- **Do I Feel Unworthy?**
    - Work on self-worth (see Chapter 17) to accept that you do deserve good outcomes.
- **How Can I Reach Out for Support?**
    - If you feel yourself sliding into sabotage, tell a mentor or counselor. Often, naming the behavior aloud stops it from escalating.

Allow yourself to enjoy and build on success rather than tear it down.

---

12. Celebrating Others' Success During Your Own Struggles

If a friend or relative is doing really well—getting a great job, buying a house, or starting a family—while you still struggle, jealousy or bitterness might arise. This can deepen your sense of "I am always behind." Instead, try:

- **Genuine Congratulation**
    - Show happiness for them, even if it stings a bit. This fosters good relationships and might lead them to help you more if they can.
- **Ask for Tips**
    - Politely ask, "How did you manage that? Any advice for me?" You might learn helpful strategies.
- **Focus on Your Path**
    - Their success does not mean you cannot succeed too. Life is not a single-lane race. Your time to flourish can come as well.

Avoid letting others' achievements drag you into self-pity. Instead, see them as proof that progress is possible.

---

13. Handling Triggers That Remind You of Prison

Sometimes, a low moment arises because you are reminded of prison life—maybe through a certain sound, smell, or authority figure. These reminders can spark fear, anger, or sadness. Quick tips:

- **Grounding Techniques**
    - Focus on the present by naming objects around you or feeling your feet on the ground.
- **Positive Affirmation**
    - Remind yourself, "I am free now, and I have choices."
- **Seek a Safe Person or Place**
    - If possible, step away from the trigger and call or visit someone who understands.
- **Long-Term Desensitization**
    - Over time, face mild triggers while practicing calm responses. This can reduce their power.

Triggers might never go away fully, but they can lose their intensity as you learn to cope (see also Chapter 12 for more on this).

---

14. Learning to Adapt Without Losing Your Values

When life hits you with big changes, you might have to adapt routines, jobs, or living situations. Just be sure you do not lose sight of your core values—like honesty, kindness, or legality. For instance:

- **If You Need Quick Money**
    - Do not revert to illegal hustles. Instead, look for short-term gigs or ask for help from a community program.
- **If Someone Urges You to Lie**
    - Stick to truth, even if it is difficult. Lying can unravel the trust you have built.
- **If You Feel Pressure from Old Friends**
    - Recall your reasons for staying out of crime. Adapt by finding new social circles or safe ways to keep limited contact if needed.

Change your methods, not your principles. This ensures you maintain integrity through all ups and downs.

---

15. Keeping an Eye on Warning Signs

You might sense a downturn coming by noticing certain warning signs:

- **Rising Stress**: You are snapping at people more, losing sleep, or feeling constant worry.
- **Ignoring Responsibilities**: Skipping bills or work shifts.
- **Drifting from Positive Habits**: Stopped going to meetings, dropped exercise, or lost contact with good influences.

If you spot these signs, act early. Talk to someone you trust, renew your healthy habits, or speak with a counselor. Early action is easier than waiting until a full crisis hits.

---

16. Building a Routine That Supports Stability

A stable daily or weekly routine can help smooth out the rollercoaster of ups and downs. This might include:

- **Regular Sleep Times**
    - Going to bed and waking up at consistent hours improves mood and energy.
- **Scheduled Tasks**
    - Knowing when you will job hunt, do chores, or have personal time reduces chaos.
- **Check-Ins with Support**
    - A weekly call or meetup with a mentor or group keeps you accountable and supported.
- **Personal Time for Reflection**
    - Even 10 minutes a day to sit quietly, write in a journal, or pray/meditate can help you process your emotions.

A routine does not eliminate surprises, but it gives you a sturdy framework to return to when life shakes you.

---

17. Celebrating Good Changes in a Responsible Way

When you have a real triumph—like clearing a parole condition, saving a certain amount of money, or achieving a healthy milestone—recognize it in a safe, measured manner:

- **Enjoy a Simple Reward**
    - A small meal at a favorite restaurant, a new book, or a budget-friendly day trip can feel special without wrecking finances or risking relapse.
- **Share with Close People**
    - Let them know you appreciate their support in getting you this far.
- **Plan the Next Goal**
    - Once you reach one milestone, aim for another to keep momentum going.

By using sensible ways to mark good times, you keep from going overboard or risking your progress.

---

18. Using Setbacks to Strengthen Resolve

Strange as it sounds, each low point is a chance to grow stronger. Ask yourself after a rough patch:

- **What Did I Learn?**
    - Did the setback reveal a weak point in your plan, a new trigger, or a skill you still need?
- **How Did I Handle It?**
    - If you handled it poorly, note what you would do differently next time. If you handled it well, pat yourself on the back and keep that strategy.
- **What Motivated Me to Keep Going?**
    - Identifying what pushed you to bounce back can help you use that same motivation in future struggles.

Over time, these lessons pile up, making you more adaptable and self-aware.

---

19. Staying Connected to Your Bigger Purpose

When life gets tough or too easy, do not forget the purpose you identified (see Chapter 16). Whether it is caring for family, serving a community cause, or living by a certain faith principle, that deeper reason can steady you:

- **Review It Regularly**
  - Maybe keep a small note with your purpose statement in your wallet or phone.
- **Apply It to Daily Decisions**
  - If your purpose is to be a good father, ask yourself, "Does this choice support being a good father?"
- **Talk About It**
  - Sharing your purpose with a supportive person can strengthen it. They might remind you of it when you feel lost.

Purpose acts like a compass, guiding you through both sunshine and storms.

---

20. Conclusion of Chapter 18

Coping with life's ups and downs is a core skill for any man rebuilding life after prison. Each day can bring new challenges or joys. Recognize that these fluctuations are normal—success does not mean everything will stay perfect forever, and a setback does not mean you should give up. By celebrating small progress, preparing for and learning from setbacks, and keeping a balanced view, you maintain steady momentum.

A strong support system, healthy routines, and safe coping methods can protect you during the worst lows and keep you grounded during the best highs. Stay mindful of warning signs that you might be drifting toward crisis or self-sabotage, and act early to correct your path. Above all, remember why you are working so hard—your purpose, your family, your freedom, or whatever inspires you deep inside. When the ride gets bumpy, that reason can anchor you until the road smooths out again.

Life after prison is not about erasing the dips completely, but about learning to manage them in a way that does not derail your progress. With practice, you will find that each time you get back up after a setback, you add another layer of resilience to your character. Over time, those layers build a future where the ups can be enjoyed more fully and the downs are handled with confidence and hope.

Chapter 19: Planning for a Better Future

Moving forward after prison is not just about fixing day-to-day problems. It is also about mapping out a clearer future. A good plan gives you direction so that you do not get stuck in the same routines or fall into old traps. Planning for a better future does not require fancy talk or perfect circumstances. It just takes honest thinking about what you want, what you need, and how to step toward those goals.

In this chapter, we will look at how to define your future aims in detail, gather the tools you need, and organize tasks so they feel less overwhelming. You will learn how to spot risks before they become disasters, how to use your strengths in new ways, and how to keep yourself motivated when the next steps seem far off. Even if you start small, having a practical plan can change everything about how you approach each day.

---

1. Why Planning Matters So Much

When you left prison, you might have felt like you were dropped into the deep end. Suddenly, you have to handle housing, money, relationships, work, and legal conditions, all at once. Without a plan, it is easy to become scattered, reacting to every little crisis or impulse. A plan brings order. It shows which tasks need immediate focus and which can wait. It also sets a roadmap for longer-term aims, such as saving up, learning a trade, or reuniting with family.

A simple but real benefit: When you create a plan, you give yourself reasons to say "no" to temptations. If your plan is to stay out of certain risky neighborhoods or avoid certain old friends, then you already have a guide in place. If your plan is to save $500 to get a better apartment, you remind yourself not to waste money on quick thrills. Planning grounds your actions in a bigger picture, so you are less likely to drift back to old ways.

---

2. Defining Your Future Aims

It is not enough to say "I want a better life." That is too vague. Your mind needs specifics so you can build a path. Think about the following areas:

- **Career or Work**: Do you want a stable, full-time job in a particular field? A short-term gig that grows into something else? Do you want to learn a skilled trade?
- **Education**: Do you need a GED or wish to attend a vocational school? Are there certificates you can earn that boost your chances in the job market?
- **Family or Relationships**: Do you want to repair a relationship with a parent, sibling, or child? Maybe have a more peaceful home environment or become a better partner?
- **Financial Goals**: How much do you want to save in the next 6 months or a year? Do you have debts you aim to reduce?
- **Housing**: Is there a safer or more comfortable place you dream of renting or owning in the future?
- **Health and Well-Being**: Do you want to reach a certain fitness level, deal with a medical issue, or manage stress more effectively?

Writing these aims down is crucial. Try to be as detailed as possible without feeling intimidated. Even if an aim seems far off, put it on paper. You are allowed to dream about a future that is different from your past, as long as you keep your feet on the ground for daily steps.

---

3. Breaking Down Big Goals into Practical Steps

Say you have a big aim like, "I want to start my own small landscaping business." That can feel enormous if you only see the end result. The trick is to break it into smaller tasks:

1. **Research**: Look up licenses or permits needed in your area. Learn the basic tools required.
2. **Save Money**: Figure out how much you need to buy or rent the necessary equipment.
3. **Get Experience**: If you can, try working for someone else's landscaping company first to see the day-to-day reality.
4. **Build a Client List**: Start by offering small services to neighbors or friends.
5. **Set a Launch Date**: Decide on a rough time—maybe 6 months to a year from now—when you want to start operating officially.

These steps turn a large dream into bite-sized pieces. After you finish one step, move to the next. If a step proves harder than expected, you can revise your plan, but you still have direction.

4. Checking What Resources You Have

People often think they have nothing, but that is rarely true. Resources can be:

- **Personal Skills**: Are you good at talking to people, fixing things, organizing tasks, or working outdoors?
- **Supportive People**: Friends, family, mentors, or counselors who can guide you, recommend you to employers, or just encourage you.
- **Community Programs**: Nonprofits or government offices that offer job training, housing referrals, or small loans.
- **Online Tools**: Free tutorials on websites that teach trades, budgeting, or even basic math and writing.

List out your resources. Many men overlook what is already in front of them. For instance, you might have a friend who knows someone in construction and can connect you to day labor. Or you might have a free community library where you can study for a GED. By mapping out resources, you see the practical help available to carry out your plan.

5. Identifying Your Gaps

Once you see your aims and resources, figure out what you are missing:

- **Skill Gaps**: Maybe you need basic computer skills to apply for certain jobs. Perhaps you need better reading comprehension to pass a license exam.
- **Financial Gaps**: You might need an initial sum to buy tools, pay for a course, or cover deposit fees for housing.
- **Document Gaps**: Some goals require IDs, birth certificates, or other legal papers. If you do not have them, you need to request or replace them.
- **Network Gaps**: If you want to start a business but do not know anyone who does that work, you may need to find a mentor or join a local business group.

These gaps are not reasons to give up. They are simply issues to address. You can add tasks to your plan like, "Sign up for a free computer class," or "Apply for a small grant at the nonprofit center." Each gap has potential solutions if you look carefully.

---

6. Creating Timelines and Deadlines

Having a wish or a "someday" plan can lead to endless procrastination. Instead, assign rough deadlines. For instance:

- By the end of this month, collect the forms needed to get your driver's license back.
- In three months, sign up for a vocational course.
- Within six months, have at least $300 in savings.
- One year from now, apply for advanced job positions or consider part-time business ventures.

These deadlines do not have to be perfect. Life might force you to adjust them. But a target date pushes you to act instead of waiting for the "right time." Checking these dates regularly also helps you see if you are falling behind, so you can re-strategize.

---

7. Dealing with Old Triggers and Bad Influences

A realistic future plan must include how to avoid falling back into the patterns that got you locked up. If certain individuals or places led you to crime, how will you stay away or limit contact? If substance use was an issue, how will you manage urges or stress in safer ways?

- **Set Boundaries**: Make a clear decision about who or what is off-limits if it threatens your plan. That might mean blocking phone numbers of certain associates or not visiting certain neighborhoods.
- **Have a Backup**: If you find yourself stuck around a risky situation (for instance, a cousin who deals drugs), who can you call or where can you go to remove yourself quickly?
- **Use Accountability**: Tell a trusted friend or mentor about your triggers, so they can warn you if they see you slipping.

Your plan should protect your freedom and progress. Sacrificing old ties or habits might be painful, but it is better than risking your future for people or lifestyles that only drag you back.

---

8. Keeping Motivation Alive

Even with a plan, motivation can fade. You might run into setbacks like rejection letters, slow progress, or discouraging people. To keep going:

- **Review Your "Why"**: Remember why this plan matters. Maybe you want a secure home for your child, or you never want to see the inside of a prison cell again.
- **Mark Smaller Wins**: Each time you complete a step—like opening a bank account or finishing a course—recognize that you are moving forward.
- **Update Your Plan**: If you learn about a better route, do not be scared to revise your steps. This is not quitting; it is adapting to new info.
- **Have Inspirational Reminders**: Some people keep quotes or photos of loved ones where they can see them. Even a sticky note on your mirror can remind you of your ultimate goal.

Motivation is not constant. But consistent small efforts, even on days you feel lazy, eventually add up to bigger results.

---

9. Finding Mentors or Role Models

If you know someone who has walked a similar path—maybe another formerly incarcerated person who is now doing well—that person can guide you. Mentors show you what steps they took, how they handled setbacks, and how they overcame doubt. If you do not know anyone personally, look around:

- **Local Reentry Groups**: They might have volunteers or staff who have been in your shoes.
- **Community Centers**: Sometimes retired workers or professionals volunteer as mentors.
- **Workplace**: A supervisor or coworker might offer good advice if you show genuine interest.
- **Online Videos or Stories**: Be careful on the internet, but you can find positive talks from people who have turned their lives around.

A good mentor does not fix your life for you. They share knowledge, cheer you on, and hold you accountable. Finding even one person who believes in your plan can boost your chances significantly.

---

10. Addressing Legal or Administrative Barriers

Your plan might involve dealing with parole requirements, old warrants, or fines. Tackle these systematically:

- **List All Obligations**: Note your parole meeting dates, court appointments, or restitution payments.
- **Schedule**: Mark them on a calendar. Missing a court date or appointment can ruin your progress.
- **Get Clarifications**: If something is unclear, contact your parole officer or a legal aid service. Do not guess.
- **Track Payments**: If you owe fines or child support, keep careful records of each payment. This proves you are meeting your obligations.

Clearing or reducing legal barriers might take time, but it is worth it. Each completed requirement is one less obstacle in your future. By staying organized and proactive, you show officials you are serious about changing.

---

11. Making Your Plan Visible

A plan hidden in your mind can be forgotten easily. Write it out. Use a notebook, a phone app, or even a poster on your wall. Include:

1. **Goals** (short-term and long-term).
2. **Steps** (broken down into tasks with target dates).
3. **Resources** (people, programs, notes about contacts or websites).
4. **Checkpoints** (when you will review progress).

Glance at it often. Update it as you move forward. If you are worried about privacy, keep it in a locked drawer or a password-protected file. But do not rely on memory alone. Seeing it in plain sight can remind you daily of what you need to do next.

---

12. Budgeting for Your Plan

Many future aims require money—whether for training, housing deposits, or just stable living. A budget (see Chapter 13) is part of the plan. Decide how much you can set aside each week or month for your goals. For example:

- **If You Need $500 for a Car Down Payment**: How many months will it take if you save $25 a week?
- **If a Trade Course Costs $400**: Could you pay $100 a month for four months? Could you find a low-cost or free version of that course somewhere else?

Thinking about money early prevents surprises. If you see a shortfall, you might look for part-time gigs or day labor to speed up savings. Or you might cut back on non-essentials for a while. Having clear numbers gives you control.

---

13. Balancing Immediate Tasks and Long-Term Vision

It is easy to get stuck focusing on immediate tasks like paying rent and meeting parole checks. These tasks are urgent, of course, but do not forget your bigger vision. If your long-term dream is to become a skilled welder, keep reading or practicing whenever you can, even if you are currently flipping burgers to pay bills.

Set aside specific hours each week for future-focused efforts. Maybe you read welding manuals online or watch tutorial videos. Or you shadow a neighbor who welds as a hobby. Over time, these small efforts bring your dream closer, even if your daily job is not glamorous. Balancing the urgent and the long-term is part of a mature plan.

---

14. Creating a Risk Management Strategy

Plans can derail if you ignore possible hazards. Think about what might threaten your plan:

- **Health Issues**: If you have a chronic condition or a history of mental health challenges, how will you maintain treatment or checkups?
- **Legal Surprises**: Are there any pending cases or fines that could pop up?

- **Bad Habits**: Do you have a pattern of quitting when stressed, or turning to quick fixes like gambling or substance use?
- **Unstable Relationships**: Could a toxic partner or friend sabotage your progress?

List these risks and outline how you will handle them. For example, if you might be tempted to drink when stressed, plan an alternative coping method (like exercise or calling a support person). This does not remove every danger, but it keeps you alert and ready to respond instead of being caught off guard.

---

15. Having a Backup or Emergency Fund

We mentioned budgeting, but it helps to mention an emergency stash again. Even $200 set aside can reduce panic if your car breaks down or you lose a part-time job. That small cushion can keep you from feeling forced to do something illegal for quick cash. Aim to build it slowly. Put a little aside each time you get paid, even if it is only $5. Over months, it grows. That money can protect your plan from being derailed by sudden problems.

---

16. Evaluating Your Plan Regularly

Situations change—maybe you find a better opportunity than the one you first aimed for, or you discover that your timeline was too tight. Set a habit of reviewing your plan:

- **Monthly Check**: Look at your goals, deadlines, and progress.
- **Ask Questions**: Am I on track? Did I miss any steps? Are my resources still available? Do I need new training or new contacts?
- **Stay Flexible**: If you see a better approach, modify your plan rather than forcing the old route. Adaptation is a sign of growth, not failure.

This helps you keep the plan alive, rather than letting it become a forgotten document.

17. Handling Doubt or Criticism About Your Plan

Some people may dismiss your future aims, saying "You are a dreamer," or "No one will hire you with a record." Do not let their negativity define what is possible. Still, it is wise to consider if they have any valid points. For example, if they say you lack certain credentials, maybe that is an area to work on. But if they are simply being harsh, trust your research and keep going.

Also watch out for self-doubt. If you feel overwhelmed, break the plan into even smaller steps or seek advice from someone you trust. Doubt is normal when aiming high, but taking consistent action is what counts.

---

18. Learning to Negotiate and Compromise

Sometimes, your plan involves other people—like a landlord, employer, or family member. You might not get exactly what you want. Learn to negotiate:

- **Explain Your Goals Clearly**: If you want a landlord to give you a chance despite a record, highlight your steady income and references.
- **Offer Solutions**: Maybe propose a slightly higher deposit or an extra letter of recommendation.
- **Stay Polite**: Even if they resist at first, keep your tone calm. Show them you are serious.
- **Be Open to Adjustments**: If they ask for something in return (like seeing consistent pay stubs for a few months), see if that is doable.

Negotiation is part of building a future. Sometimes you do not get an immediate "yes," but you create a path forward by showing willingness to meet halfway.

---

19. Building Patience for Long-Term Gains

Many men get frustrated when big results do not come fast. Prison might have taught you to respond to things instantly. The outside world's success stories—like owning a home or mastering a job skill—often take time, sometimes years. Cultivate patience:

- **Focus on the Next Step**: Instead of obsessing over how far away your end goal is, do the next small step well.

- **Compare to Your Past**: Notice how far you have already come since your release. Maybe you used to have no stable place to stay, and now you have a small but steady room. That is progress.
- **Avoid Quick Scams**: If something promises instant riches or success, it is probably dangerous or fake. Real growth takes effort and time.

Patience does not mean laziness. It means steady, consistent action without expecting overnight miracles.

---

20. Conclusion of Chapter 19

Planning for a better future after prison is about more than just wishing. It is about turning hopes into a step-by-step layout of what you want, what you have, and what you need to do. By writing down specific goals, breaking them into tasks, and setting deadlines, you give yourself a structure that steadies you against day-to-day chaos. You also develop a sense of purpose that makes it easier to avoid old patterns and temptations.

Of course, no plan is flawless. You might face setbacks, unexpected changes, or criticism from people who doubt you. That is normal. The real power of a plan is that it can adapt. If one path closes, you find another. If you learn a better method, you revise your approach. Along the way, you can keep your eyes on the bigger picture—like staying free, building a stable life, and becoming someone you can respect when you look in the mirror.

When planning feels tough, remember your reasons for starting this journey. Think about the life you do not want to return to, and the life you hope to have. Each step, however small, carries you closer to that vision. Combine your resources, manage your risks, and keep updating your plan as you grow. Over time, the results will speak for themselves: more security, more respect (both from others and from yourself), and a path that leads far away from the mistakes that once confined you.

Chapter 20: Keeping Up Your Progress for Years to Come

You have put in the effort to reenter society, handle daily struggles, and maybe even reach some of your initial goals. But the work does not end when you secure a job or fix relationships. The real question is how to maintain this progress over the long haul. Many men do well for a few months or a year, only to slide back into harmful habits or lose steam when life throws bigger challenges.

This final chapter tackles how to stay on track years from now, not just in the first phase of reentry. It will explore ways to keep learning, continue improving your environment, nurture healthy relationships, and stay mentally strong so that you do not slowly drift back toward behaviors that could wreck your freedom again. By planning for the long term, you give yourself the best chance at a lifetime of stability and growth.

---

1. Viewing Change as a Lifelong Process

It is common to see reentry as a single phase—get out of prison, find a job, follow parole rules. But real transformation continues beyond that. In reality:

- **Habits Need Ongoing Care**: Even if you have avoided old vices for a year, you still need to be mindful. New stresses can tempt you to return to what is familiar.
- **Goals Evolve**: Once you achieve an initial aim (like finishing parole or saving some money), you will want bigger or different goals to stay motivated.
- **People Change**: Friends, family, or mentors might move on or face new situations. You will need fresh support networks or new ways to adapt.

Embracing a mindset of continual learning and adjusting keeps you from thinking, "I am done. I can relax now." While you do deserve rest and a sense of accomplishment, do not let that slip into complacency.

---

2. Building a Routine of Self-Improvement

If you rest on your successes, you might stagnate. A routine of self-improvement can be simple but steady:

- **Read or Study Regularly**: If you have a library card or internet access, explore books, articles, or tutorials. Keep your mind active.
- **Set Yearly or Seasonal Goals**: Each year, decide on new skills, certifications, or personal changes you aim to accomplish.
- **Attend Workshops or Groups**: Local community centers often have free or low-cost seminars on everything from finance to computer literacy.
- **Track Your Progress**: Use a notebook or app to mark each step. This helps you see growth over time.

By consistently learning, you remain adaptable. You do not get stuck in the mindset of "I already learned what I need to know." The world changes, so you must keep up.

---

3. Staying Connected to Positive Communities

A big mistake is pulling away from supportive groups once you think you no longer "need" them. Those groups—whether they are faith-based, recovery-oriented, or skill-focused—often provide ongoing encouragement and accountability. If you step away, you might slowly slide back into isolation or connect with less helpful crowds.

Try to maintain membership or at least some form of regular contact. Maybe you attend once a month instead of once a week if you are busier. Keep relationships alive with people who understand your background and still push you to stay on the right path.

---

4. Periodically Checking Your Environment

As you grow, you might outgrow certain living arrangements or social circles. For instance:

- **Neighborhood Conditions**: If your area is filled with negative influences or triggers, you might consider moving, even if it takes time to save up.

- **Housemates or Roommates**: Someone who was once supportive might become a source of stress or temptation if their behavior changes.
- **Coworkers**: If your workplace environment is toxic or encourages shady behavior, you might need to look for a more honest or stable job.

Checking your environment every 6 to 12 months can help you spot red flags. If you see that your surroundings are dragging you down, you can plan an exit or upgrade. This does not happen overnight, but awareness is the first step.

---

5. Updating Your Financial Goals Over Time

Your money situation will (hopefully) improve if you keep working steadily. Once your basic needs are met—rent, food, utilities—you can tackle bigger money aims:

- **Paying Off Debt**: If you had loans, fines, or past bills, clearing them frees your future paychecks.
- **Building Emergency Savings**: Increase your safety net from $200 to $1,000, then aim for one month's living costs if possible.
- **Investing in Yourself**: Maybe you can afford better tools for a trade, a course for a certification, or a used car to expand job options.
- **Longer-Term Savings**: If you dream of owning a small home or sending a child to college, start a separate fund, even with small monthly amounts.

Regularly review these financial milestones. As you hit one, set the next. This keeps you from slipping into wasteful spending. It also gives you a sense of progress that can last for years.

---

6. Planning for Major Life Events

Over time, you might face big life changes—marriage, children, health shifts, or even caring for aging parents. Think about these possibilities:

- **Parenting**: If you plan to have children or already do, how will you be there for them consistently? Do you need better housing, a stable schedule, or counseling to handle past trauma so you can parent effectively?

- **Health Changes**: Getting older often brings new concerns. Stay on top of medical checkups. If you develop a chronic issue, adapt your work and lifestyle accordingly.
- **Retirement**: It might feel far away, but consider whether you can set aside a small amount for older age. Even a few dollars a week can grow over decades.
- **Moving**: If your job offers a chance in another city, or you want a fresh environment, how can you prepare financially and emotionally?

Being proactive means you do not scramble last-minute when these big life events arrive. You cannot predict everything, but a little thought can go a long way.

---

7. Handling Plateaus or Boredom

After a few years out of prison, you might settle into a routine—job, home, occasional hobbies. At some point, you could feel bored or unchallenged. This boredom can tempt you to take risks for excitement. Instead, find healthier ways:

- **Try New Hobbies**: You can explore sports, crafts, or community projects you never tried before.
- **Volunteer**: Helping at shelters, youth programs, or local events can give a sense of purpose beyond your daily work.
- **Mentor Others**: If you have learned a lot about reentry, you could guide people who are just getting out. Teaching them can also remind you of how far you have come.
- **Set a Big Goal**: Maybe you want to run a half marathon, write a short book, or refurbish an old car. A new challenge keeps your mind active.

Plateaus do not mean something is wrong. They are a natural pause. Use them to explore fresh territory without falling into dangerous thrills.

---

8. Dealing with Relapses or Lapses

A relapse could be returning to a substance, breaking a parole condition, or just slipping into behaviors you promised to avoid (like gambling or aggression). A lapse might not land you back in prison immediately, but it can signal a bad pattern. If this happens:

1. **Accept Responsibility Quickly**: Denying or hiding it can make things spiral out of control.
2. **Seek Support**: Reach out to a counselor, mentor, or friend who can help you analyze what led to this slip.
3. **Revisit Your Strategies**: Did you stop using your coping methods? Did you ignore a trigger?
4. **Learn From It**: A relapse can be a harsh lesson on where your plan or mindset failed.
5. **Get Back on Track**: Do not assume everything is ruined. People can and do recover from setbacks if they address them promptly.

The faster you respond to a lapse, the easier it is to contain the damage. Long-term stability often involves responding effectively to these stumbles rather than living in fear of them.

---

9. Maintaining Good Relationships

Over the years, relationships require care. If you have a partner or children, do not let daily stress overshadow their needs. Some practices:

- **Regular Communication**: Take time to talk with your partner about concerns, plans, and feelings. With children, check in about school or their activities.
- **Solve Conflicts Calmly**: If arguments arise, try to handle them with respect (see Chapter 15 on speaking clearly and listening well).
- **Create Family Traditions**: Simple weekly or monthly routines (like a shared meal, game night, or walk) keep bonds strong.
- **Apologize and Forgive**: Over the years, small grudges can grow if not addressed. Show humility when you are wrong, and do not hold onto anger if they apologize.

Healthy bonds anchor you during tough seasons. They also give you more reasons to avoid returning to crime or self-destructive actions.

10. Keeping Mental Health in Check

Your mental health can shift over time. Even if you managed stress well at first, new traumas or old buried issues might surface. Options to maintain mental balance:

- **Periodic Check-Ins with a Counselor**: Even if you only go once every few months, having a professional to talk to can catch problems early.
- **Stress-Reduction Techniques**: Keep up with physical exercise, breathing exercises, or journaling.
- **Socializing with Positive People**: Isolation can worsen anxiety or depression. Friendly contact can boost your mood.
- **Watch for Warning Signs**: If you start losing interest in daily life, or have trouble sleeping or overwhelming sadness, do not wait—get help from a mental health professional or a hotline.

Keeping your mind healthy is just as important as preventing physical harm. It affects every area of your life, from work performance to family interactions.

---

11. Exploring Deeper Meaning or Faith

Some men find that exploring spiritual or moral beliefs gives them long-term motivation to stay on the right path. Whether you follow a religious tradition or a personal moral code, having a deeper sense of meaning can bring peace and direction. If you are open to it:

- **Join a Place of Worship**: If it aligns with your views. Many offer community support, moral guidance, and volunteer activities.
- **Practice Private Reflection**: Meditation, prayer, or quiet reading can center your mind on values you want to uphold.
- **Seek Guidance**: Spiritual leaders or ethical mentors can help you think through big life questions beyond the daily grind.

You do not have to be religious to have a moral or spiritual core. The key is to connect with values that go beyond mere survival, guiding you to be a better person even when no one is watching.

---

12. Giving Back to Those in Need

Long-term growth includes helping others. This might be in the form of mentoring someone who just got out of prison, volunteering at a local shelter, or donating small amounts to causes you believe in. By contributing, you:

- **Strengthen Your Sense of Purpose**: Knowing your experience can help others makes your past less of a chain and more of a tool for good.
- **Reduce Self-Focus**: When you see other people's struggles, you appreciate what you have and stay humble.
- **Build a Legacy**: Over years, you become known not just for your past but for your positive impact.

This giving back can also protect you from slipping into old negativity. When you serve others, you keep your mind on being someone who lifts up, rather than tears down.

---

13. Handling Major Temptations Years Later

You might think that if you avoided crime or addiction for a few years, you are safe. But sometimes big temptations appear suddenly—like a friend who returns from out of town and wants you to join a shady scheme, or a stressful personal crisis that makes you crave numbness through a substance. Plan for these rare but dangerous moments:

- **Know Your Absolute Lines**: For instance, no matter how tough things get, you will not handle stolen goods or spend time with someone dealing illegal substances.
- **Have a Support Contact**: Keep at least one person you can call 24/7 in an emergency if you feel yourself slipping.
- **Practice Quick Exits**: If a place or person feels risky, leave immediately, even if it seems rude. Better a rude exit than a ruined life.
- **Remember Past Consequences**: Think back to what prison life was really like. The shock of that memory can help you say "no" to repeating mistakes.

Time does not always erase risk. Long-term stability depends on being ready for any curveball, even if it arrives years down the line.

14. Setting an Example for Younger People

As you get older, you might realize younger relatives or neighbors see you as an example. If you keep your progress going, you can show them that a record does not define a life forever. You might:

- **Share Advice**: Help them avoid the traps you fell into.
- **Model Good Work Ethic**: Let them see you handling responsibilities, paying bills, and keeping a calm home environment.
- **Encourage Their Growth**: If they want to learn a skill or find a job, guide them to resources you discovered.
- **Stay Genuine**: If you made a mistake, admit it. Show them that it is possible to correct course without shame or giving up.

By guiding others, you also keep reminding yourself of the lessons you learned, reinforcing your own commitment to a positive way of life.

---

15. Preparing for Unexpected Shifts

Life can bring random events—a serious illness, an economic downturn, a family tragedy. You cannot plan for every scenario, but you can:

- **Maintain a Network**: Keep relationships strong. People can help when big events strike.
- **Stay Flexible**: If a dream job suddenly vanishes, adapt your skills to a new field.
- **Keep Learning**: The more diverse your skillset, the easier it is to pivot if one area collapses.
- **Maintain Savings**: As best as you can, keep building that emergency fund.

When shocks happen, it might feel like you are back at square one. But if you have built resilience and a solid base over years, you will stand a better chance of bouncing back more quickly.

---

16. Avoiding Complacency

Long-term success can breed complacency. You might think, "I have been out of trouble for 5 years, so I am good now." But life is not static. You must still keep an eye on your mental state, your social circle, and your habits. Sometimes, middle-age or later-life crises can cause men to revert to reckless behavior they thought they left behind.

Check in with yourself. Ask:

- Have I become lazy in my routines or finances?
- Do I ignore possible warning signs, thinking I am above them now?
- Am I still learning, or have I stalled out?

If you see signs of slipping, take action before it becomes a bigger problem. Renew your commitments or find new goals to pursue.

---

17. Celebrating (Marking) Milestones Sensibly

When you hit 5, 10, or 20 years outside prison without legal trouble, that is a big deal. You might also mark personal milestones like paying off a large debt or buying a small house. Recognize these achievements in a way that does not risk all your progress:

- **Keep It Safe and Reasonable**: A small gathering with trusted folks, a nice meal, or a day trip to a local spot.
- **Reflect on the Journey**: Use the milestone to look back at how you grew and to thank people who helped.
- **Set New Targets**: Ask, "What is next?" so you do not end up with an empty feeling after the celebration.

Even though we avoid using a specific word for big festivities, we can still say it is good to "mark" or "acknowledge" big achievements. This helps you appreciate how far you have come and recharge for the future.

---

18. Being Open to Self-Reflection

Decades can pass since your release, and you might feel content with how things turned out. Yet, there is always room for self-reflection:

- **Check on Old Wounds**: Are there still regrets or guilt you have never addressed? Dealing with them can free you from hidden shame.

- **Revisit Family Ties**: Maybe an estranged sibling is now open to reconnecting, or you want to deepen relationships you once took for granted.
- **Examine Beliefs**: Your perspectives on morality, success, or faith might evolve. Do not be afraid to question them and grow.
- **Stay Grateful**: Reflect on the second chance you have. This fosters humility and a sense of responsibility to keep living right.

Self-reflection keeps you from becoming rigid or ignoring parts of your life that might need healing or improvement.

---

19. Sharing Your Story Responsibly

Over the years, you may find opportunities to share your experience with schools, community panels, or podcasts. If you choose to do this:

- **Focus on Lessons**: Talk about what you learned and how you changed, rather than just the sensational parts of crime or prison.
- **Keep It Honest**: Do not exaggerate or lie about your past. People value truthful accounts.
- **Respect Boundaries**: If your story involves others who prefer privacy, avoid revealing their details.
- **Have a Positive Message**: Show that change is possible, but do not pretend it is easy. Balance hope with realism.

Sharing your story can influence others for good, but do so in a way that aligns with your own well-being and respects the privacy of those involved in your past.

---

20. Conclusion of Chapter 20 (and of the Book)

Keeping up your progress for years to come means recognizing that you are on a lifelong path. Each season of your life will bring fresh challenges—aging parents, changing job markets, personal growth, or new relationships. But the foundation you have built—self-awareness, strong habits, a healthy network, and practical skills—can carry you through these changes without reverting to the mistakes that once cost you your freedom.

You have already shown, by reading and applying the lessons in these chapters, that you care about a better life. You have learned about managing anger, building self-worth, finding decent housing, getting stable work, saving money, and staying out of legal trouble. You have explored how to repair relationships, handle stress, and plan for a future that goes beyond just surviving. Now the task is to maintain and expand on all that.

Stability is not a one-time finish line but a continuing practice. You stay on guard against old triggers, keep an eye on your finances, adapt your plans as new opportunities appear, and revise goals as you grow. You also remain alert to the well-being of your mind, body, and closest connections. In the end, this kind of steady diligence is what makes the difference between someone who slips back and someone who keeps moving forward, year after year.

This book has given you a framework and many tips. The rest is in your hands. Continue to refine your skills, respect your own worth, and place yourself among people and settings that support the man you want to be. No matter how rocky the past has been, each day is another chance to add to the good you do and the legacy you leave behind. Through consistent effort and wise choices, you can remain free, stable, and genuinely proud of the life you are building—long after your prison sentence has ended.

www.ingramcontent.com/pod-product-compliance
Lightning Source LLC
LaVergne TN
LVHW012103070526
838202LV00056B/5606